DEDICATION

*This book is dedicated to
ALL my Students*

THIRD EDITION

HUMAN ANATOMY
and PHYSIOLOGY
LABORATORY MANUAL
PART II BIOL-2402

with

**PHOTO ATLAS
AND CLINICAL
APPLICATIONS**

PIUS ABOLOYE, M.D. (Dr.P)

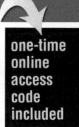

one-time
online
access
code
included

Kendall Hunt
publishing company

Cover image © Shutterstock, Inc.

Kendall Hunt
publishing company

www.kendallhunt.com
Send all inquiries to:
4050 Westmark Drive
Dubuque, IA 52004-1840

CONTENTS

PREFACE

My numerous life achievements have been possible through my faith and trust in God: for "I can do all things through Christ who strengthens me", Phil. 4:13, my parents for their discipline and guidance. For that and much more I have been blessed tremendously.

Teaching Anatomy and Physiology fell into my lap (literally) by accident, starting off as an Adjunct Faculty at Tarrant County College, then to North Lake College. I immediately found out how much I loved teaching A and P and extremely passionate about laying the foundation for success in the Medical Field for tomorrows doctors, dentists, PA's, Nurses and other Allied Health Pre-Professional students.

My sincere thanks to the Chair of our Department: Dr. Marilyn M. Mays for her vision and guidance, giving me the first opportunity to teach full time at this level. And to my colleagues and staff at North Lake for their continued support and allowing me to effectively educate our students even though sometimes we are not on the same page, my thanks.

In particular, Gabriel Bohak, many thanks for his assistance in taking some of the Laboratory Model photos with me. Best wishes to you in Medical School.

I set out to write a Lab Manual primarily for my students:

- To ease the burden of the ever increasing cost of books
- To simplify the materials without losing foundational course content
- And in the Format that I teach.

New to this Revised Edition: Added Web Companion to aid as both practice and graded exercises to reinforce key concepts.

To my students: past and present, thanks for letting me part of your educational process and for laughing at my jokes in class and your inspiration and positive feedbacks. Some of you are now my colleagues and remained in contact. To the future student(s), I hope you too would benefit from the book and my teaching style of relevant Clinical Applications to Anatomy and Physiology.

ABOUT THE AUTHOR

PIUS A. ABOLOYE, M.D, received his Medical Degree from Meharry Medical College in Nashville, Tennessee, trained in General Surgery (Trauma) at the University of Texas Health Sciences Center, San Antonio Texas and worked at JPS Hospital in Fort Worth, Texas for several years prior to teaching. He started his medical career at the same hospital as a Pharmacist before going to Medical School.

Dr. P, as he is affectionately known by his students has been teaching Human Anatomy and Physiology for over 10 years, most of those at North Lake College. In addition he has taught Pharmacology and Pathophysiology at other area and local Colleges and Universities.

He created, developed and continued to teach the ALL Online and Blended (Hybrid) Format Anatomy and Physiology Courses (in addition to Regular Courses) at North Lake College.

Interests: Dr. P is passionate about his family, kids, and Volunteering—he goes on Medical Missions every year to Central and South Americas and the Philippines. While he enjoys cycling and jogging, his other passion is Wine Tasting!

Special Senses

Upon completion of this exercise, you should be able to:

A. Locate and identify the structure of the human eye.
B. Locate and define the functions of the extrinsic muscles of the eye.
C. Identify the accessory structures of the eye.
D. Trace the pathway of vision with the structures involved.
E. Locate and identify the structure of the human ear.
F. Trace the pathway of sound with the structures involved.
G. List the clinical applications on special senses.

NEEDED MATERIALS

1. Human Eye Model plus photo atlas/diagram.
2. Human Ear Model plus photo atlas/diagram.
3. Ear ossicles (3).
4. Bony labyrinth (cochlear).

Introduction

I. OVERVIEW

A. Special senses include vision, hearing and balance, smell, and taste.
B. The eye and the ear are the largest in the class. The human ear houses two organs (cochlea and vestibule) for hearing and balancing, respectively.
C. Located within each of these organs are specialized receptors, retinal rods and cones in the eye, hairy cells, and organ of corti in the ear. They receive and transmit the information on the respective nerves (optic, vestibulocochlear) to the appropriate cerebral cortices for interpretation.

II. EYE: ANATOMY

A.

TABLE 13-1 Eye Structures (Intrinsic)

STRUCTURE	DEFINITION/FEATURES
TUNICS (3)	
■ **SCLERA**	Outer fibrous coat. Anteriorly becomes the cornea. At the junction of the sclera and cornea is the sclera-venous sinus for the drainage of aqueous humor.
■ **CHOROID**	The vascular tunic would become modified anteriorly into 3 structures: ciliary body, the iris (pigmented portion), and suspensory ligament, responsible for accommodation.
■ **RETINA**	The neural tunic has the photoreceptors (rods, cones).
CORNEA	The transparent layer of the eye; is a continuation of the sclera. Also known as "window of the eye" and helps focus light into the lens.
IRIS	An extension of the ciliary body anteriorly and partially in front of the lens, leaving a gap called the pupil. The pupil regulates the amount of light into the eye.
SUSPENSORY LIGA-MENT	Also an extension of the ciliary body; holds the lens. Contraction or relaxation of the ciliary body and the ligaments changes the lens shape and light accommodation.
MACULA LUTEA	"Yellow spot" on the retina and within it is the fovea centralis, highest density of cone receptors.
FOVEA CENTRALIS	Fovea ("depression/indent") is located within the macula lutea. Has the highest density of cone receptors.
OPTIC DISC	This is where the optic nerve exists in the eyeball. Lack any photoreceptors. Also known as "blind spot" in visual fields where both eyes overlap.
OPTIC NERVE	Cranial nerve II, are axons of the ganglion cells of the retina leading away from the eyeball toward the cerebral visual cortex.
VITREOUS HUMOR	This is the content of region behind the lens, also called the posterior cavity. Made of semisolid material, keeps the eyeball from collapsing, lasts a lifetime.
AQUEOUS HUMOR	This is the content of the region behind the cornea and in front of the lens, also called the anterior cavity. Made of watery material, continuously secreted and reabsorbed via the Canal of Schlemm. Its overproduction or inadequate drainage can cause glaucoma.
SCLERAL-VENOUS SINUS	Also known as "Canal of Schlemm," located at the transition junction of the scleral and the cornea anteriorly. Drains the aqueous humor.
LENS	Avascular hard biconvex structure. Its shape can be adjusted (flattened or rounded) by the ciliary body (and suspensory ligaments) to accommodate more or less light and focus it on the retina.
CILIARY BODY	A continuation of the vascular tunic (choroid) anteriorly. Ciliary body becomes 2 structures: iris (pigmented portion) and the ciliary zonule (suspensory ligaments) that holds the lens. Autonomic changes (sympathetic/parasympathetic) stimulate the ciliary body and therefore change the shape of the lens (light control) and the iris (diameter of the pupil).
PUPIL	The center diameter of the pigmented iris in front of the lens, it is regulated by the autonomic nervous system.
ORA SERRATA	This is the anterior border of the retina where the choroid layer is exposed. Appears jagged edge ("serrated knife").

B.

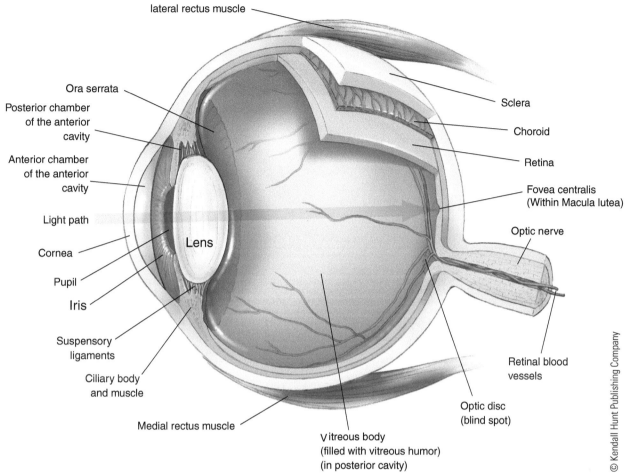

FIGURE 13-1 Sagittal View Anatomy of the Human Eye

C. ACCESORY EYE STRUCTURES

I)

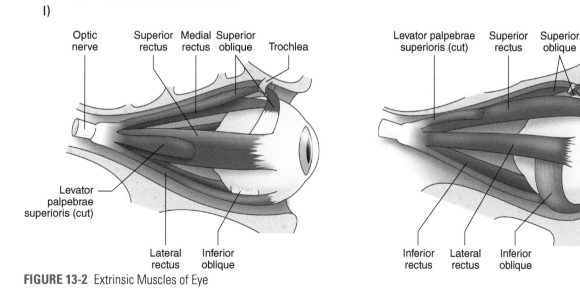

FIGURE 13-2 Extrinsic Muscles of Eye

II)

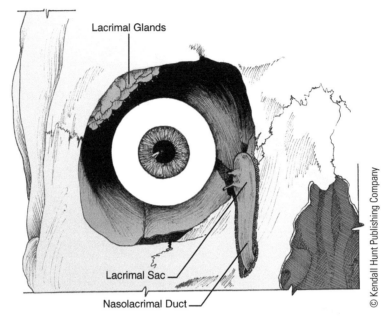

FIGURE 13-3 Lacrimal Gland Eye

III)

TABLE 13-2 **Muscles of the Eye**

MUSCLE	FUNCTION	CONTROLLING CRANIAL NERVE
SUPERIOR RECTUS	Moves eye superiorly	Oculomotor III
INFERIOR RECTUS	Moves eye inferiorly	Oculomotor III
MEDIAL RECTUS	Moves eye medially	Oculomotor III
LATERAL RECTUS	Moves eye laterally	Abducen VI
SUPERIOR OBLIQUE	Moves eye inferiorly and laterally	Trochlea IV
INFERIOR OBLIQUE	Moves eye superiorly and laterally	Oculomotor III

IV)

TABLE 13-3 **Eye Structures (Extrinsic)**

STRUCTURE	DEFINITION/FEATURES
EYEBROWS	Along with eyelashes, they protect the eye from foreign objects and act as partial shades. Eyelashes are short hairs at the free borders of each eyelid.
EYELIDS	Upper and lower folds of skin-covered muscles protect the eyeball. It is lined by the thin moist conjunctiva.
CONJUCTIVA	The mucous membrane lining the inner eyelids ("whites of the eye"); it is a continuation of the sclera anteriorly. Jaundice is "yellow conjunctiva."
LACRIMAL APPARATUS	
▪ **LACRIMAL GLAND**	Located on the superior lateral aspect, produces tears to lubricate the eye. Tear contains water and lysozyme enzyme (antibacterial).
▪ **NASOLACRIMAL DUCT**	Drains tears from the lacrimal sac via the lacrimal canal and empties to the roof of the nose.

D. Lab Activity 13-1: Identify the Structures on the Eye Model and Photo/Atlas

LIST OF TERMINOLOGY: Eye Structures

EYE	STRUCTURES	EXTRINSIC EYE MUSCLES
sclera	canal of Schlemm	superior rectus
choroid	pupil	inferior rectus
retina	conjunctiva	lateral rectus
cornea	lacrimal gland	medial rectus
iris	lacrimal puncta	superior oblique
optic nerve, chiasm and track (visual pathway)	lacrimal ducts (superior and inferior)	inferior oblique
suspensory ligament	lacrimal sac	
macula lutea	nasolacrimal duct	
fovea centralis		
optic disc		
vitreous body		
aqueous humor		
lens		
ciliary body		

E. VISUAL PATHWAYS:

HUMAN EYE ANATOMY
THE RETINA

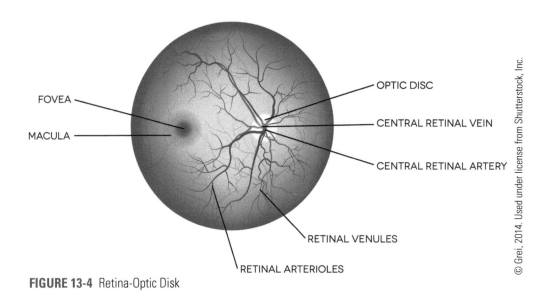

FOVEA

MACULA

OPTIC DISC

CENTRAL RETINAL VEIN

CENTRAL RETINAL ARTERY

RETINAL VENULES

RETINAL ARTERIOLES

© Grei, 2014. Used under license from Shutterstock, Inc.

FIGURE 13-4 Retina-Optic Disk

The Visual Projection Pathway

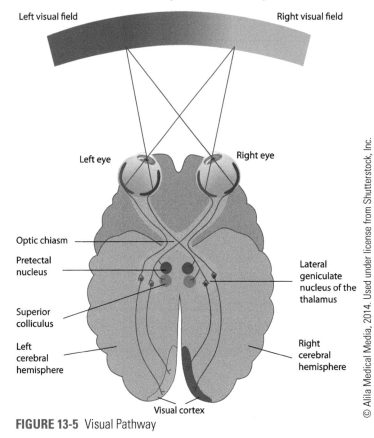

Left visual field

Right visual field

Left eye

Right eye

Optic chiasm

Pretectal nucleus

Superior colliculus

Left cerebral hemisphere

Lateral geniculate nucleus of the thalamus

Right cerebral hemisphere

Visual cortex

© Alila Medical Media, 2014. Used under license from Shutterstock, Inc.

FIGURE 13-5 Visual Pathway

F. Lab Actvity 13-2: Dissection of the Cow Eye

EXAMINE STRUCTURES IN A COW EYE	
1.	Obtain a preserved cow eye and your dissecting instruments.
2.	Examine the external anatomy of the eye. Note specifically the sclera, cornea, and optic nerve. The eye may still retain a cushion of adipose tissue that protects the eye in the orbit of the skull.
3.	Trim away any adipose tissue. Using scissors, make an incision slightly lateral to the cornea, and continue cutting around the cornea to remove it from the eyeball. (Photo 376a)
4.	The black pigmented area surrounding the lens is the ciliary body. Can you detect the suspensory ligaments attaching the lens to the ciliary body?
5.	The pupil is the hole in the center of the iris, which is a continuation of the ciliary body.
6.	Carefully remove the lens from the eyeball. Note its consistency.
7.	The vitreous humor within the posterior compartment is a viscous fluid that amplifies the image and helps the eyeball to retain its shape.
8.	The retina is a shiny membrane on the inner surface of the posterior compartment. Find the macula lutea and the optic disc.
9.	When you have completed your examination of the eyeball, discard it in the bag provided.

III. Ear: Anatomy

A.

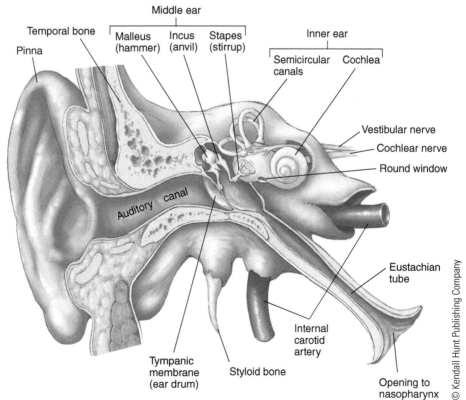

FIGURE 13-6 Sagittal View Anatomy of the Human Ear

B.

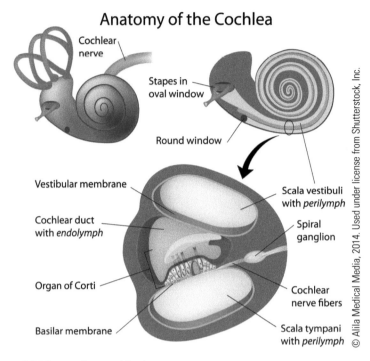

Anatomy of the Cochlea

Cochlear nerve

Stapes in oval window

Round window

Vestibular membrane

Scala vestibuli with *perilymph*

Cochlear duct with *endolymph*

Spiral ganglion

Organ of Corti

Cochlear nerve fibers

Basilar membrane

Scala tympani with *perilymph*

© Alila Medical Media, 2014. Used under license from Shutterstock, Inc.

FIGURE 13-7 Organ of Corti

C.

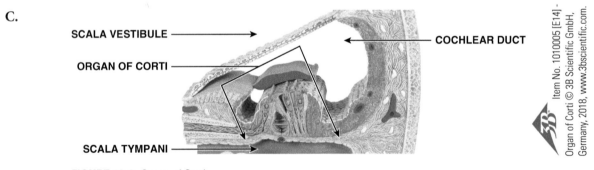

SCALA VESTIBULE

COCHLEAR DUCT

ORGAN OF CORTI

SCALA TYMPANI

Item No. 1010005 [E14] - Organ of Corti © 3B Scientific GmbH, Germany, 2018, www.3bscientific.com.

FIGURE 13-8 Organ of Corti

D. Lab Activity 13-3: Identify the Structures on the Ear Model and Photo/Atlas

LIST OF TERMINOLOGY: Ear Structures

Auricle (pinna)	Oval window
external acoustic meatus	round window
tympanic membrane	**cochlea**
Ossicles: malleus, incus, stapes	■ cochlear duct
eustachian tube	■ organ of Corti
osseous labyrinth	■ tectorial membrane
membranous labyrinth	**vestibular apparatus:**
endolymph, perilymph	■ vestibule
	■ semicircular canals

E.

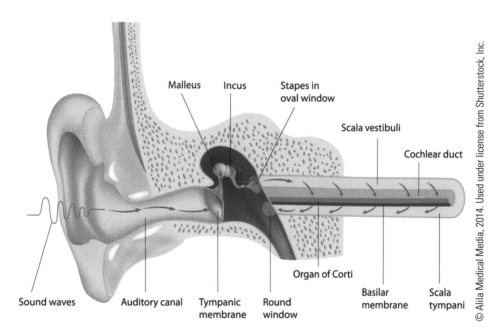

FIGURE 13-8A Auditory Pathway

IV. Clinical Applications: Diseases of Special Senses

TABLE 13-4 Clinical Applications on Special Senses

DISEASE/CONDITION	DEFINITION/FEATURES
CONJUCTIVITIS	Inflammation of the visible sclera (whites) or conjunctiva. Manifests itself with redness, irritation, and photophobia. May be bacterial, viral, or congenital conjunctivitis in the newborn second to maternal sexually transmitted infection.
GLAUCOMA	Chronic increase of pressure in the anterior chamber in front of the lens. May be caused by increased aqueous humor fluid production or failure to drain (at Canal of Schlemm).
CATARACT	Increased cloudiness of the lens resulting in decreased vision or loss of vision (blindness). Unknown etiology/causes, but may be due to toxins, aging, trauma, or diabetes.
DEAFNESS	Loss of hearing (partial or total).
■ **CONDUCTION**	Anything that blocks the transmission of pathway of sound but before the Organ of Corti.
■ **SENSORINEURON**	Anything that damages the transmission at the Organ of Corti (hair cells) and the auditory nerve pathway of sound up to and including auditory cortex.
MACULA DEGENERATION	Decreased vision or acute loss of vision; both eyes are typically involved. Central vision is affected, while peripheral vision remains intact.
MINERRE SYNDROME	Complex of symptoms involving both organs in the bony labyrinth (cochlear for hearing and vestibule for balance). Patient presents with hearing loss, syncopy, and nausea/vomiting.
EXTERNAL OTITIS	Also called "swimmers ear." Inflammation of the external auditory canal second to bacteria/fungi infection from contaminated pools. Manifests itself with fever, pain, itching, and hearing loss (often temporarily).
OTITIS MEDIA	Middle ear infection common in 6 to 24-month-old children. Second to bacterial infection from the naso- or oropharynx that ascends into the Eustachian tube. Manifests itself with fever, pain, itching and pulling of ear, and hearing loss (is often temporarily).
STRABISMUS	May be caused by extraocular muscle defect, corneal opacities, retinal disease, or refractive index error. The result is deviation of eyes.
ASTIGMATISM	Unknown causes. Irregular cornea or lens leads to uneven focus of images and hence decreased vision.
MYOPIA	Abnormal configuration leads to convergence of light in front of the retina. There's decreased acuity for distant objects.
HYPEROPIA	Usually second to age. There's decreased acuity for near objects. Abnormal configuration leads to convergence of light in behind the retina.
DIABETIC RETINOPATHY	Decreased or loss of vision second to diabetes mellitus. Damage to retinal vessels.

A. Answer the following:

1. The outer visible lining of the human eye is the called:

   A. anterior chamber

   B. conjunctiva

   C. cornea

   D. iris

2. The iris is what type of muscle?

   A. skeletal

   B. smooth

   C. cardiac

3. The balance and equilibrium senses are both located in the:

   A. inner ear

   B. middle ear

   C. oval window

   D. outer ear

4. The posterior eye chamber made up of thick, gel-like is called the

   A. vitreous humor

   B. endolymph

   C. perilymph

   D. aqueous humor

5. The pigmented part of the eye is also called:

   A. conjunctiva

   B. iris

   C. cornea

   D. pupil

6. The external auditory meatus/canal ends at the level of:

   A. cochlea

   B. vestibule

   C. oval window

   D. tympanic membrane

7. Damage to the right lateral rectus muscle on the right side would deviate the right eye to what direction?

   A. laterally

   B. medially

   C. superiorly

   D. inferiorly

8. The auditory hair cells are located in:

   A. organ or corti

   B. ampullae

   C. maculae

   D. saccule

9. The iris is a continuation of this tunic:

   A. sclera

   B. retina

   C. choroid

   D. eyelid

10. The area of highest acuity (photoreceptors) is the:

    A. sclera

    B. retina

    C. fovea

    D. choroid

11. Describe the structures in the middle ear.

12. Describe the structures in the inner ear.

13. Why do infants commonly have otitis media (middle ear infection) than adults?

14. Describe the causes of the two major classes of deafness (conduction and neuronal).

15. Describe the function of the eustachian tube.

V. Post-Lab Activity 13-4: Use the Eye and Ear Models and Photo/Atlas/Diagrams

A) Locate and Identify these structures

I)

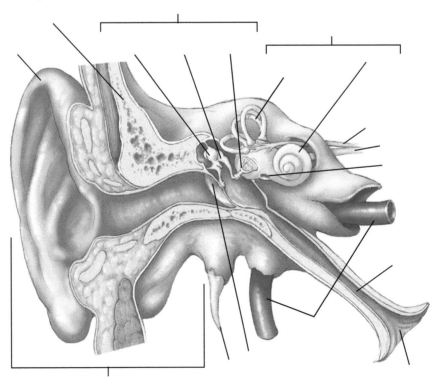

FIGURE 13-9 Sagittal View Anatomy of the Human Ear

II)

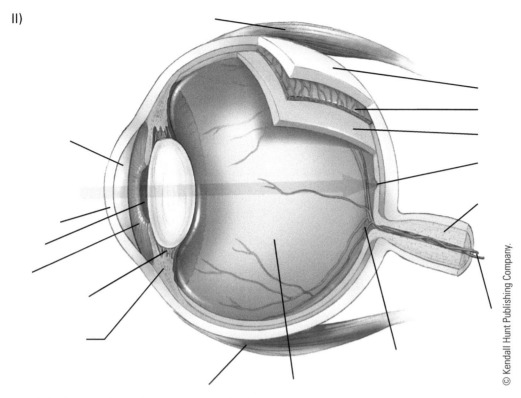

FIGURE 13-10 Sagittal View Anatomy of the Human Eye

Endocrine System

LEARNING OUTCOMES

Upon completion of this exercise, you should be able to:

A. Identify the locations and microscopic features of the major endocrine organs.
B. Describe the function(s) of the endocrine system.
C. List the endocrine organ, its hormone(s), target tissues, and the hormone(s) actions(s).
D. Define negative and positive feedback in the controlling hormone release.
E. Describe the locations of and the anatomical relationships between the hypothalamus, anterior pituitary, and posterior pituitary glands.
F. Explain the role of the hypothalamus in the release of anterior and posterior pituitary hormones.
G. Name other endocrine organs, their hormones, and actions.
H. List the clinical applications on endocrine conditions and diseases.

NEEDED MATERIALS

1. Human torso
2. Models: Human brain (full and mid-sagittal section), larynx (with thyroid gland), pancreas, and kidney (with adrenal glands) models.
3. Male and female reproductive organs.
4. Microscope slides: pituitary, thyroid, thymus, adrenal, pancreas, ovary, and testis.

Introduction

I. OVERVIEW

A. The endocrine system includes the following major organs: hypothalamus, pituitary, pineal, thyroid, parathyroid, thymus, adrenals, pancreas, testes, and ovaries.
   Other hormone-producing glands/organs include placenta, heart, kidney, and skin.

B.

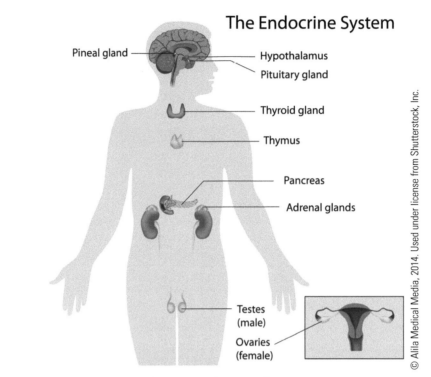

FIGURE 14-1 Major Organs of the Endocrine System

C. Negative vs. Positive Feedback Control

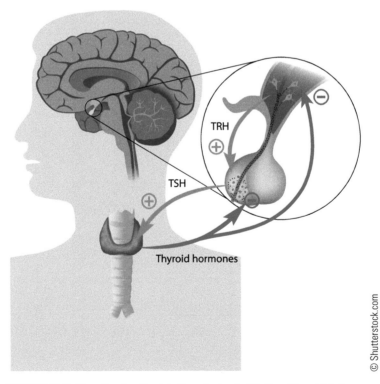

FIGURE 14-2 Negative Feedback in Hypothalamic-Pituitary-Thyroid Axis

D. **FEATURES:** The endocrine system performs multiple functions including the following:
   1. Maintaining homeostasis
   2. Endocrine and nervous systems compared

TABLE 14-1A Endocrine Versus Nervous System Compared

FEATURED CHARACTERISTICS	ENDOCRINE SYSTEM	NERVOUS SYSTEM
BASIC FUNCTION(S)	Maintain homeostasis and communication.	Maintain homeostasis and communication.
REACTION TIME TO STIMULI	Slow.	Fast.
DURATION OF RESPONSE OR EFFECT	Long.	Short.
ADAPTATION TO PROLONGED STIMULI	Slow.	Fast.
TARGET TISSUES	Widespread, all body tissues.	Specific muscles and glands.
CHEMICAL MESSENGER(S)	Hormones.	Neurotransmitters.
MESSENGER-PRODUCING CELLS	Endocrine glands (cells).	Neurons.
DISTANCE OF MESSENGER TO TARGET TISSUES		Short (at synaptic clefts).
ADAPTATION TO PROLONGED STIMULI	Slow.	Fast.
MESSENGER(S) OVERLAP FUNCTIONS	Some hormones function as neurotransmitters.	Some neurotransmitters function as hormones.
TARGET TISSUES OVERLAP	Have receptors on similar organs/tissues.	Have receptors on similar organs/tissues.

E. Lab Activity 14-1: Identify these Endocrine Structures on the Brain, Larynx, Human Torso, and Reproductive Models

See Photo Atlas

LIST OF TERMINOLOGY: Endocrine organs:

- hypothalamus
- pituitary gland
- pineal gland
- thyroid gland
- parathyroid glands
- pancreas
- adrenal (supra-renal) glands
- testes
- ovaries

II. The Hypothalamus with Pituitary Relationship and Pineal Gland

A1.

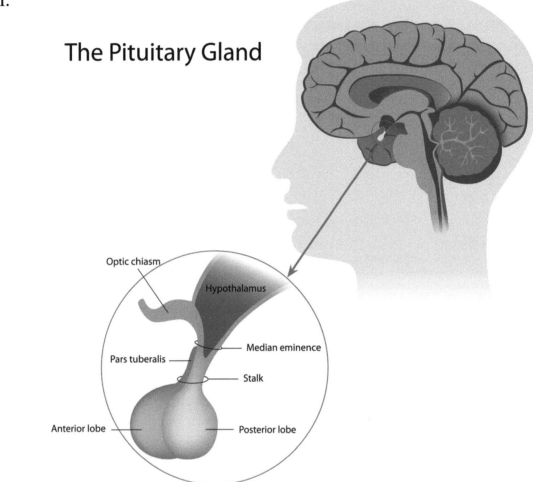

The Pituitary Gland

FIGURE 14-3 The Pituitary Gland

A2.

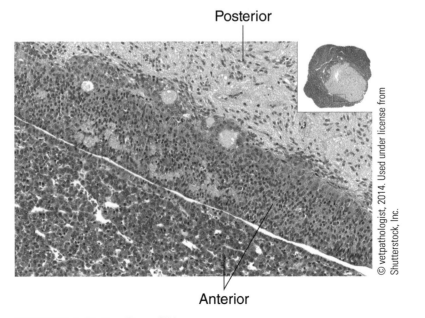

FIGURE 14-4 Pituitary Tissue Slide

B.

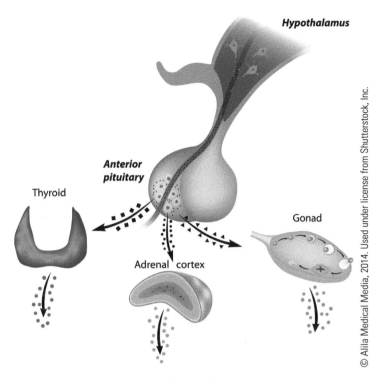

FIGURE 14-5 The Hypothalamic Pituitary Organ Axes

C.

TABLE 14-1 Hypothalamus–Pituitary Hormones

GLAND	HORMONE	TARGET	ACTION
HYPOTHALAMUS	Thyrotropin-releasing hormone **(TRH)**	Anterior pituitary gland	Release of **TSH**
	Corticotropin-releasing hormone **(CRH)**		Release of **ACTH**
	Gonadotropin-releasing hormone **(GnRH)**		Release of gonadotropins **(FSH and LH)**
	Prolactin-releasing hormone **(PRH)**		Stimulates release of **prolactin**
	Prolactin-inhibiting hormone **(PIH)**		Inhibits the release of **prolactin**
PITUITARY (ANTERIOR LOBE)	Growth hormone **(GH)**	All body cells	Stimulates growth (bone, muscle)
	Thyroid-stimulating hormone **(TSH)**	Thyroid gland	Development and activity of thyroid
	Adrenocorticotropic hormone **(ACTH)**	Adrenal cortex	Release of glucocorticoids by adrenal gland
	Follicle-stimulating hormone **(FSH)**	Reproductive organs	Gamete formation
	Luteinizing hormone **(LH)**	Reproductive organs	Production of gonadal hormones
	Prolactin **(PRL)**	Mammary tissue	Stimulates milk production

(continued)

TABLE 14-1 Hypothalamus–Pituitary Hormones (*continued*)

GLAND	HORMONE	TARGET	ACTION
PITUITARY (POSTERIOR LOBE)	Oxytocin	Uterus and breast	1. Stimulates uterine contractions 2. Stimulates milk ejection (letdown)
	Antidiuretic hormone (ADH)	Renal tubules	Reabsorption of water (results in decreased urine output and increased blood volume)

i) HYPOTHALAMIC-HYPOPHYSEAL PORTAL SYSTEM: Network of blood vessels transports hormones between the hypothalamus, pituitary stalk, pituitary, and the systemic blood.

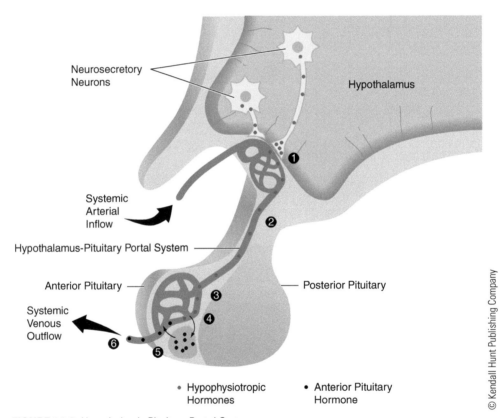

FIGURE 14-6 Hypothalamic Pituitary Portal System

ii) POSTERIOR PITUITARY

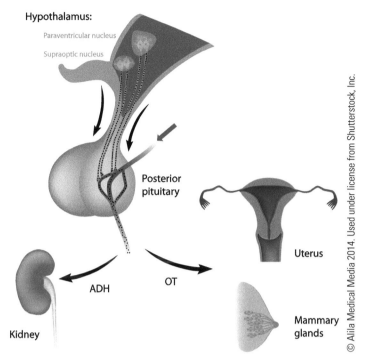

FIGURE 14-7 Hypothalamic Pituitary Portal System

D. PINEAL GLAND: Located in the posterior section of the diencephalon, produces melatonin believed to be associated with mood and sleep–awake cycle.

E. Lab Activity 14-2: Identify the Structures on the Brain Models

See Photo Atlas

LIST OF TERMINOLOGY:

- hypothalamus
- pituitary gland
- pineal gland
- pituitary tissue slide (view)

III. Thyroid and Parathyroid Glands

A1.

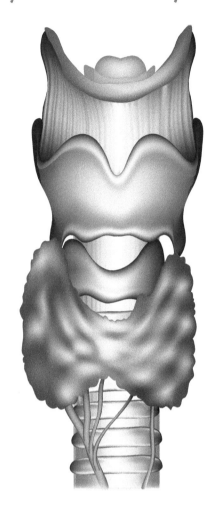

A2.

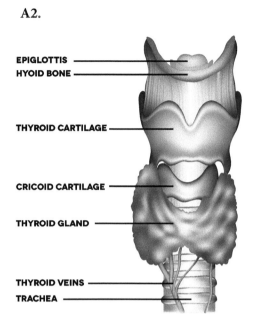

THYROID GLAND

FIGURE 14-8 Anatomy of Thyroid gland, Epiglottis, Trachea

A. See FIG 14-2 Negative Feedback in Hypothalamic-Pituitary-Thyroid Axis

B.

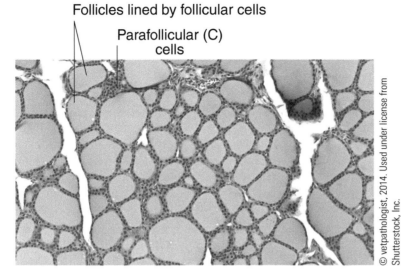

Follicles lined by follicular cells

Parafollicular (C) cells

© vetpathologist, 2014. Used under license from Shutterstock, Inc.

FIGURE 14-9 Thyroid Tissue Slide

C.

TABLE 14-2 Thyroid and Parathyroid Hormones

GLAND	HORMONE	TARGET	ACTION
THYROID	Thyroid hormone **(TH)** ■ T_3 and T_4 ■ **T_3** is the most effective/preferred by cells. ■ **T_4** is the most abundant in plasma. ■ T_3 or T_4 is easily interconverted to the other.	All cells	Increases cellular metabolism (oxygen consumption and heat production) in most cells.
	Calcitonin.	Bone, kidney, GI tract	Decreases blood calcium levels. Increases osteoblast activity.
PARATHYROID	Parathyroid hormone **(PTH)** parathormone.	Bone, kidney, GI tract	Increases blood calcium levels. Increases osteoclast activity.

D.

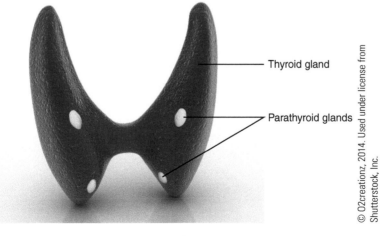

Thyroid gland

Parathyroid glands

© O2creationz, 2014. Used under license from Shutterstock, Inc.

FIGURE 14-10 Endocrine Parathyroid Gland

E. Lab Activity 14-3: Identify Thyroid and Parathyroid Glands on the Larynx Model and View Tissues Slides

See Photo Atlas

LIST OF TERMINOLOGY:

- thyroid gland
- parathyroid glands
- thyroid tissue slide (view)
- parathyroid tissue slide (view)
- thymus tissue slide

IV. Pancreas

A.

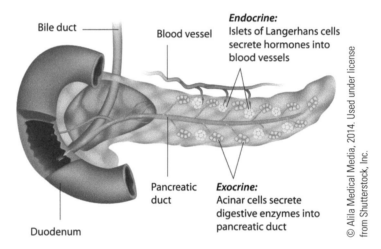

Bile duct

Blood vessel

Endocrine:
Islets of Langerhans cells secrete hormones into blood vessels

Pancreatic duct

Exocrine:
Acinar cells secrete digestive enzymes into pancreatic duct

Duodenum

© Alila Medical Media, 2014. Used under license from Shutterstock, Inc.

FIGURE 14-11 Exocrine and Endocrine Pancreas

B.

Acini   Islets of Langerhan

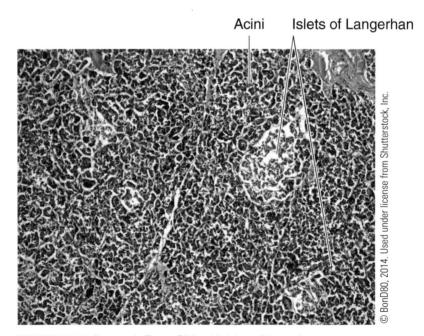

© BonD80, 2014. Used under license from Shutterstock, Inc.

FIGURE 14-12 Pancreatic Tissue Slide with Islets of Langerhans

C.

TABLE 14-3 Pancreatic Gland Hormones

CELL TYPE	HORMONE	TARGET	ACTION
BETA	Insulin	Most tissues	Decreases blood sugar by increasing reabsorption of glucose, amino acids post-digestion, resulting in glycogenesis, lipogenesis, and protein synthesis.
ALPHA	Glucagon	Liver and skeletal muscle	Increases breakdown of glycogen (glycogenolysis) and lipolysis, resulting in increasing blood sugar.

D. Lab Activity 14-4: Identify the Structures on the Pancreas Model and Tissues Slides

See Photo Atlas

LIST OF TERMINOLOGY:

- pancreas
- pancreas tissue slide (view)

V. Adrenal Glands

LIST OF TERMINOLOGY:

- suprarenal (adrenal) gland
- adrenal tissue slide (view)

A.

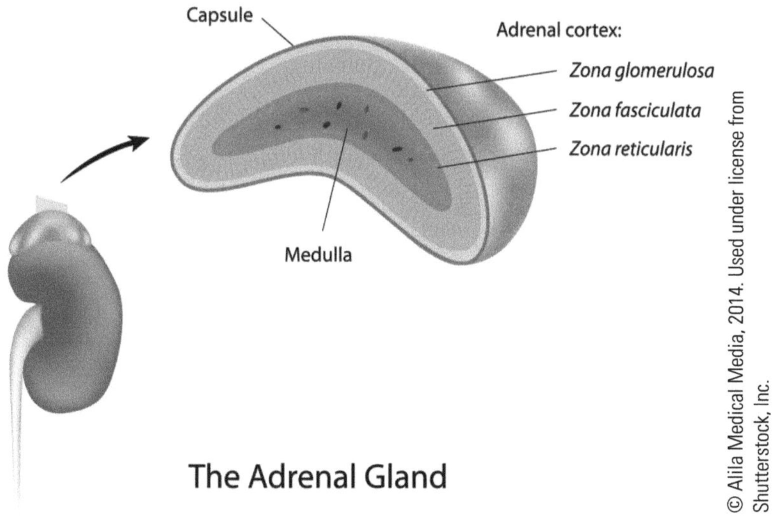

The Adrenal Gland

FIGURE 14-13 The Adrenal Gland

B.

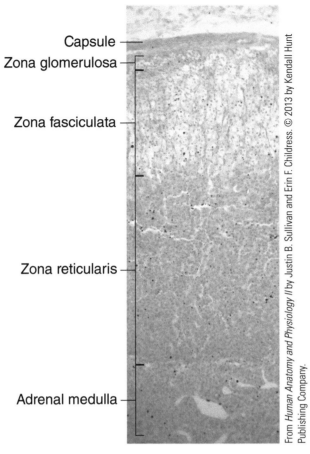

Capsule

Zona glomerulosa

Zona fasciculata

Zona reticularis

Adrenal medulla

From *Human Anatomy and Physiology II* by Justin B. Sullivan and Erin F. Childress. © 2013 by Kendall Hunt Publishing Company.

FIGURE 14-14 Adrenal Tissue Slide

C.

TABLE 14-4 Adrenal Gland Hormones

LAYER	HORMONE	TARGET	ACTION
Adrenal cortex: Glomerular layer	Mineralocorticoids (primarily aldosterone)	Renal tubule cells	Increases renal reabsorption of Na⁺ (and excretion of K⁺), hence increased blood sodium levels (indirectly water follows). Maintains blood volume in low blood pressure.
Adrenal cortex: Fascicular layer	Glucocorticoids (primarily cortisol)	Most tissue cells	Considered hormone of chronic stress. Resist stressors by increasing blood glucose, fatty acid and amino acid levels, and blood pressure. High levels depress the immune system and inflammatory response. Can cause brittle bone by increasing osteoclast activity.
Adrenal cortex: Reticular layer	Gonadocorticoids (primarily androgens)	Most tissue cells	Enhances masculine characteristics (especially in females). May be involved in sex drive.
Adrenal medulla	Catecholamines (epinephrine and norepinephrine)	Most tissue cells	Hormone of acute stress. Increases sympathetic response to stress.

D. Lab Activity 14-5: Identify the Structures on the Male and Female Models and View Tissue Slides

See Photo Atlas

VI. Testis and Ovarian (Gonadal) Hormones

A.

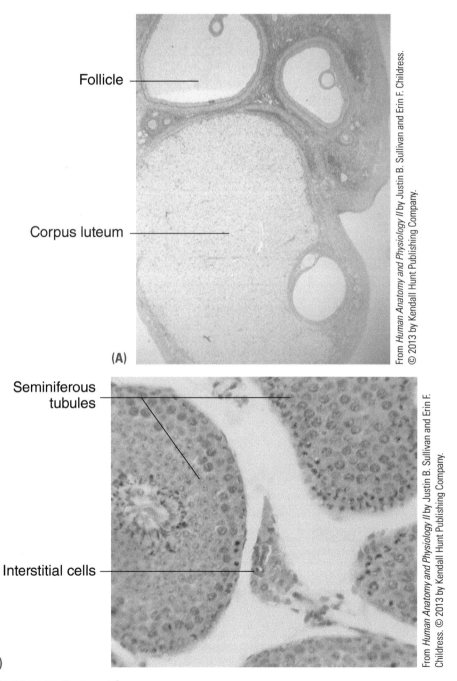

FIGURE 14-15 Testis and Ovary

B.

Seminiferous tubules

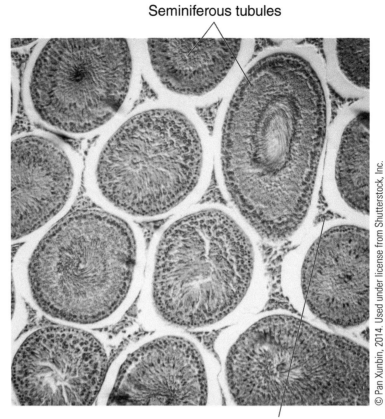

© Pan Xunbin, 2014. Used under license from Shutterstock, Inc.

Interstitial cells of Leydig

FIGURE 14-16 Testis Tissue Slide

C.

TABLE 14-5 Hormones of the Gonads

GLAND	HORMONE	TARGET	ACTION
OVARY	ESTROGEN Produced by the developing secondary follicular cells and Graafian follicle.	Female reproductive organs and breasts	Stimulate maturation and development of female reproductive system and secondary sexual characteristics.
OVARY	PROGESTERONE Produced primarily by corpus luteum.	Female reproductive organs	Action is to establish menstrual cycle in conjunction with estrogen.
TESTIS	TESTOSTERONE Produced by interstitial cells of Leydig.	Male reproductive organs	Promotes maturation of male reproductive system, the development of secondary sexual characteristics, and production of sperm gamete.

D. Lab Activity 14-5: Identify the Structures on the Male and Female Models and View Tissue Slides

See Photo Atlas

LIST OF TERMINOLOGY:

- testis
- ovary
- testis tissue slide (view)
- ovary tissue slide (view)

VII. Other Endocrine Organs/Glands

A.

TABLE 14-6 Other Endocrine Gland/Tissues

GLAND/TISSUES	HORMONE	TARGET	ACTION
ATRIAL (HEART)	ATRIAL NATURETIC PEPTIDE (ANP)	Renal tubules	Release by atrial wall is stimulated by increased blood volume returning to the atrial (in elevated BP). Increases Na+ excretion (water follows) to decrease blood volume/BP.
THYMUS	THYMOSIN THYMOPOETIN	T-Lymphocytes (immature)	T-Lymphocyte maturation in immunity.
KIDNEY	■ ERYTHROPOEITIN	Bone marrow	Produced by the JG granular cells (afferent arterioles) in response to low volume or BP or anemia. Stimulates increased red blood cell synthesis.
	■ VITAMIN D	Bone/Kidney/GI	Reabsorption of calcium and phosphate.
PLACENTA	■ hCG	Corpus luteum	Maintains the corpus luteum.
	■ ESTROGEN	Uterus/Breast	Myometrium growth and breast growth.
	■ PROGESTERONE	Uterus	↓ Uterine contraction
	■ PLACENTA LACTOGEN	Breast	↑ Mammary gland development

B.

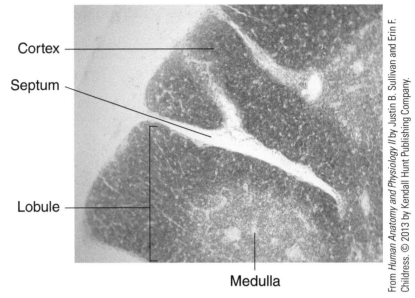

Cortex

Septum

Lobule

Medulla

FIGURE 14-17 Thymus Tissue Slide

VIII. Clinical Applications: Diseases of the Endocrine System

TABLE 14-7 Clinical Application—Diseases in Endocrine System

GLAND	DISEASE/CONDITION	PATHOLOGY	SIGNS/SYMPTOMS
PITUITARY	**GIGANTISM**	↑ Elevated growth hormone in childhood	Excessively tall height.
	ACROMEGALY	↑ Elevated growth hormone in adults	Enlarged hand, feet, face, and jaw protrusion.
	PITUITARY DWARFISM	↓ Growth hormone	Slow growth. Normal mental but slow sexual development.
	PANHYPOPITUITARISM	No hormones	Lack of endocrine activities.
	SIADH (SYNDROME OF INAPPROPRIATE ADH SECRETION)	↑ ADH	Oliguria, anuria. Generalized edema.
	DIABETES INSIPIDUS	↓ ADH often second to head trauma/ ischemia	Polyuria, polydipsia.
THYROID	**GRAVES DISEASE (MOST COMMON TYPE OF HYPERTHYROIDISM)**	↑ T3 or T4 second autoimmune disease. Hyperthyroidism	Enlarged neck, difficulty swallowing.

GLAND	DISEASE/CONDITION	PATHOLOGY	SIGNS/SYMPTOMS
	MYXEDEMA	↓ T3 or T4 second autoimmune disease, radiation/surgery. Hypothyroidism	Edema, weight gain, velvety dry skin, always cold.
	HASHIMOTO DISEASE (MOST COMMON TYPE OF MYXEDEMA)	↓ T3 or T4 second autoimmune disease. Hypothyroidism	Edema, weight gain, velvety dry skin, always cold.
	CRETINISM	↓ Congenital absence of T3 or T4	Mental retardation, poor growth.
	ENDEMIC GOITERS	↓ T3, T4, second lack of iodine. Hypothyroidism	Enlarged neck, difficulty swallowing.
PARATHYROID	HYPERPARATHYROIDISM	↑ PTH second to tumor	Weak bones, easy fractures, kidney stones.
	HYPOPARATHYROIDISM	↓ PTH often second to thyroidectomy	Overexcited neuro- and muscular system, tetany and spasm.
ADRENAL CORTEX	CUSHING DISEASE	↑ Cortisol second tumor	Hyperglycemia, diabetes, moon face, buffalo hump, stretch marks (striae).
	CONN DISEASE	↑ Aldosterone second tumor	Water retention, polydipsia, polyuria, and hypertension.
	ADDISON DISEASE	↓ Cortisol (± aldosterone), second infection or diseases	Muscle weakness, salt craving, depression, low BP.
ADRENAL MEDULLA	PHEOCHROMOCYTOMA	↑ Catecholamines (epinephrine)	↑ BP, heart rate persistently, or intermittently.
PANCREAS	DIABETES MELLITUS TYPE I (IDDM)	↓ Or No insulin second autoimmune destruction of B cells	Hyperglycemia, polyuria, polydipsia, polyphagia with weight loss.
	DIABETES MELLITUS TYPE II (NIDDM)	↓ Insulin or ↑ tissue (receptor) resistance to insulin	Often obese. Hyperglycemia, polyuria, polydipsia, polyphagia.
	DIABETIC COMA (Diabetic Ketoacidosis—DKA)	↓ Insulin levels and low blood sugar	Ketosis, acidosis, dehydration, acetone breath, drowsiness, lethargy.
	INSULIN SHOCK	↑ Insulin level	Syncopy, perspiration, trembling.

IX. Post-Lab Activity: Endocrine System Label these Structures

A.

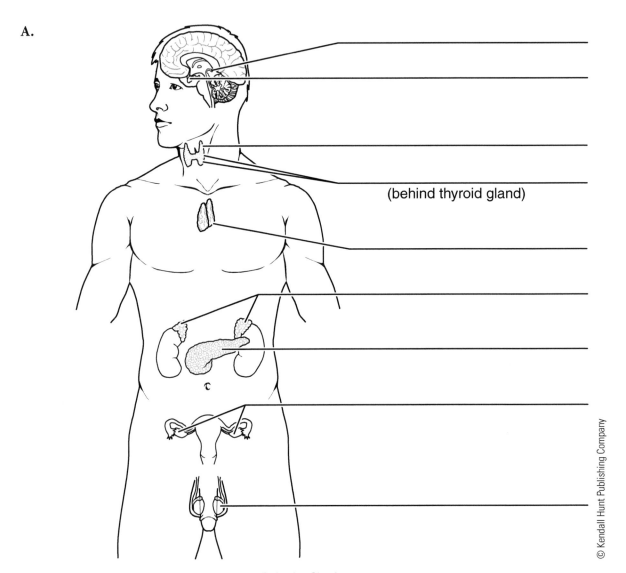

(behind thyroid gland)

FIGURE 14-18 Locate and Identify the Endocrine Glands

B. PHOTO ATLAS

C.   1. Study the thyroid gland under the microscope. Note the spherical follicles, which contain pink thyroglobulin (primarily thyroxine attached to a carrier protein). Cuboidal cells form the walls of the follicles and secrete thyroxine. Cells located between the follicles secrete calcitonin. Sketch the tyroid tissue and indicate which cells secrete thyroxine and calcitonin.

2. Study the pancreas under the microscope and sketch what you see. Notice that the islets of Langerhans are easily distinguished from the more typical cuboidal cells that form the tubes and secrete enzymes. Label an islet of Langerhans and indicate that it secretes insulin and glucagon. Label on of the non-islet tubular structures as an acinus and indicate that it secretes digestive enzymes.

3. Carefully study the summary of the endocrine system at the end of this exercise. Consider that material as being the bare minimum to be learned about the specific endocrine glands and their products. Complete the following assignment after having studied the summary.

A. Match the following target organs to the appropriate hormone:

Column A	Column B
A. Adrenal cortex	_____ 1. ADH
B. Lymphoid tissue	_____ 2. Thymosin
C. Mammary glands	_____ 3. Prolactin
D. Thyroid gland	_____ 4. TSH
E. Tubules of kidney	_____ 5. ACTH

B. Match the gland with the hormone it releases:

Column A	Column B
A. ADH	_____ 1. Anterior pituitary
B. Cortisol	_____ 2. Posterior pituitary
C. Epinephrine	_____ 3. Thyroid
D. Estrogen	_____ 4. Parathyroid
E. Growth hormone	_____ 5. Adrenal cortex
F. Insulin	_____ 6. Adrenal medulla
G. Melatonin	_____ 7. Pancreas
H. PTH	_____ 8. Testis
I. Testosterone	_____ 9. Ovary
J. Thymosin	_____ 10. Thymus
K. Thyroxin	_____ 11. Pineal gland

C. State the causes of the following endocrine disorders. Use the second line following each disorder to add any notes given by the instructor.

1. Acromegaly _____

_____

2. Dwarfism _____

_____

3. Giantism _____

_____

4. Conn's Disease _____

_____

5. Cretinism _____

_____

6. Graves' disease _____

_____

7. Myxedema _____

_____

8. Addision's disease _____

_____

9. Cushing's disease _____

_____

10. Precocity and virilism _____

_____

11. Diabetes insipidus _____

_____

12. Diabetes mellitus _____

_____

D. Answer the following questions:

1. The posterior pituitary gland secretes
   A. ADH
   B. TSH
   C. LH
   D. ACTH

2. The zona glomerulosa of the adrenal cortex produces which of these:
   A. glucocorticoids
   B. epinephrine
   C. norepinephrine
   D. mineralocorticoids

3. The action of the parathyroid hormone includes all of the following, except :
   A. increase urine formation
   B. stimulate osteoblast activity
   C. inhibit osteoblast activity
   D. stimulate osteoclast activity

4. Name the hormones causing a fall in blood sugar.
   A. aldosterone
   B. cortisol
   C. glucagon
   D. insulin

5. Which of the following is a/are hormones of the adrenal medulla?
   A. epinephrine
   B. aldosterone
   C. norepinephrine
   D. insulin

6. Calcitonin is secreted by this gland:
    A. heart
    B. liver
    C. pituitary gland
    D. thyroid gland

7. The major hormone of the corpus luteum is:
    A. progesterone
    B. cortisone
    C. aldosterone
    D. testosterone

8. This hypothalamic hormone has an effect on the uterus
    A. TSH
    B. LH
    C. oxytocin
    D. ACTH

9. Describe the endocrine functions of the pancreas.

10. Distinguish between Type I and Type II diabetes.

11. Define diabetes insipidus.

12. Name the hormones and functions of the three layers of the adrenal cortex.

13. Distinguish between hypo- and hyperthyroidism.

14. Define the role of erythropoietin.

Cardiovascular System: Blood

LEARNING OUTCOMES

Upon completion of this exercise, you should be able to:

A. Describe the major functions of Blood.
B. List blood composition.
C. List and identify the types of leukocytes, their function, and relative abundance.
D. Identify anemia (sickle cell) and leukemia slides.
E. List the clinical applications.

NEEDED MATERIALS

1. Slides: Blood smear (Wright).
2. Slides: Sickle cell anemia, infectious mononucleosis, eosinophilia, lymphocytic leukemia.
3. Blood typing kit.

Introduction

I. OVERVIEW

A. Blood components include the following:
   i) **Plasma:** Liquid portion contains water, clotting factors, plasma proteins (albumin, globulin), lipids, electrolytes, oxygen, hormones, salt, nutrients, waste, and other dissolved or suspended in fluid.
   ii) **Formed Elements: The cellular component** includes:
     a) Erythrocytes (red blood cells)
     b) Leukocytes (white blood cells)
     c) Thrombocytes (platelets)
B. **FUNCTIONS:** Blood performs multiple functions including the following:
   1. Transport of nutrients: gases, hormones, waste products, and clotting factors.
   2. Regulatory functions: temperature control, homeostasis fluid balance, blood loss prevention (coagulation by the platelets), and maintenance of osmolarity and pH.
   3. Defense: Phagocytic and immune function is performed by the white elements (leukocytes).

TABLE 15-1 Features and Functions of Blood Components

COMPONENTS	FEATURES	FUNCTIONS
RBCs	**Erythrocytes** are biconcave most numerous of the blood elements 4–5 millions.	Gas transport (O_2 and CO_2).
PLATELETS	**Thrombocytes** are fragmented cells from megakaryocytes. Second most common of the blood elements.	Forms platelet plug in clot formation to prevent leaks from damaged vessels.
WBCS	**Leukocytes.** There are 5 types divided into 2 subdivisions: **Granulocytes** (cytoplasmic granules) and **Agranulocytes** (no cytoplasmic granules).	Defense.
■ GRANULOCYTES	Has cytoplasmic granules.	
■ NEUTROPHILS	Polymorphonuclear nuclei. 3–5 segmented nuclei.	Phagocytosis.
■ EOSINOPHILS	Bilobed nuclei with orange-red-tinged cytoplasmic granules.	Allergic reactions and parasitic infection.
■ BASOPHILS	Dark blue large (indistinct) nucleus with granules.	Allergic reactions.
■ AGRANULOCYTES	Have no cytoplasmic granules.	
■ MONOCYTES	Kidney-shaped nucleus. Are macrophages.	Phagocytosis.
■ LYMPHOCYTES	Large single nucleus with just a rim of cytoplasm left.	Immunity.
● B CELLS		Antibody production in humoral immunity.
● T CELLS		Cell-mediated immunity.
PLASMA	Whole blood minus cells. Liquid portion of blood. Makes up 45–55% of blood volume. Consist of water (90%), dissolved solutes: plasma protein, clotting factors, gases, amino acids electrolytes, and wastes.	Transport and solvent.
SERUM	Whole blood minus cells and clotting factors.	Transport and solvent.

II. Lab Activity 15-1: Identify Blood Elements on Microscope

See Photos Atlas

> LIST OF TERMINOLOGY:
> - erythrocytes (red blood cells)
> - leukocytes (white blood cells)
> - thrombocytes (platelets)
> - neutrophil
> - basophil
> - eosinophil
> - monocytes
> - lymphocytes
> - anemia
> - sickle cell anemia
> - plasma

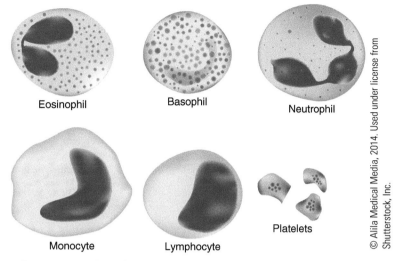

FIGURE 15-1–6 Blood Elements

III. Typing for ABO and Rh Blood Groups

A.

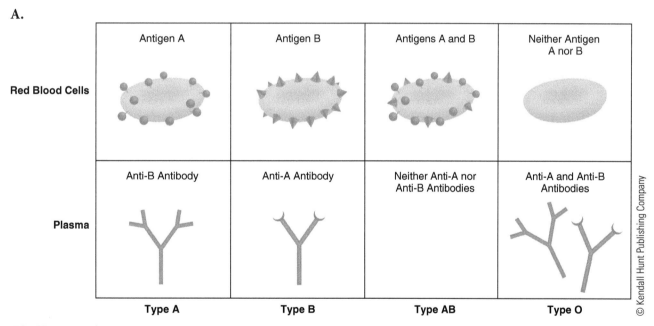

FIGURE 15-7 ABO Blood Typing

B.

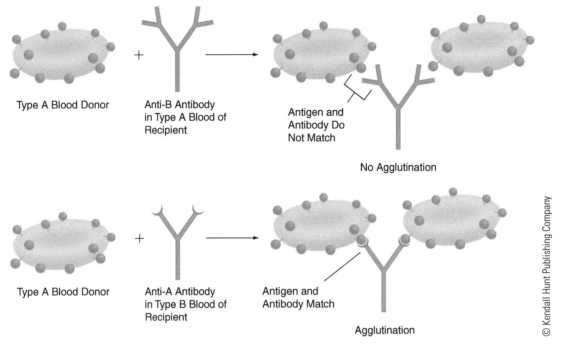

Type A Blood Donor + Anti-B Antibody in Type A Blood of Recipient → Antigen and Antibody Do Not Match

No Agglutination

Type A Blood Donor + Anti-A Antibody in Type B Blood of Recipient → Antigen and Antibody Match

Agglutination

FIGURE 15-8 ABO Blood Transfusion Reaction

C. LAB ACTVITY 15-2: Blood Typing Instructions (Know Your Blood Type):

- Each one of us need to determine his or her own blood type. The **ABO group** is the most widely used along with the Rh grouping. Knowing your blood type may prevent you from getting wrong blood transfusion and save your life.

- **Antigens (agglutinogens)** are protein surface makers on the RBC membranes, and are genetically determined. There are only two antigens: A (A blood type) or B (B blood type), or AB combination or NO antigen present (O blood type).

- **Antibodies (agglutinins):** are found in the person's plasma. Your body produces antibody to the corresponding **MISSING** antigen.

- **Rh:** another marker is also present on the RBC membrane in addition to ABO. If present, he/she is Rh+ (90% of US population); if absent he/she is Rh−. Rh− mother with an Rh+ fetus can become synthesized (at first pregnancy). Upon subsequent exposure (second and third pregnancies), she would clump/destroy the fetal blood (erythroblastosis fetalis).

- **Materials:** Blood typing kit, pencil marker, clean slide, staining tray, Antisera (A, B, and anti-Rh (D)), gloves, alcohol wipe, a lancet, tooth picks, and band aid.

  - **Follow these blood typing instructions:**

    • Divide the slide into three sections (A, B, and D) with the pencil marker. Place the slide atop the staining tray.

    • Wash and dry your hand. Wear a glove on your knife/lancet holding hand. Pin-prick your other finger with the lancet.

    • Use a pipette to pick one or two drops of blood, place the drop on Section A of the slide. Repeat the same for B and D sections.

    • Add a drop of anti-sera A onto your Section A slide. Immediately, using a toothpick gently mix these two and WAIT 3 minutes.

    • Repeat above process using anti-sera B and D onto your Sections B and D on the slide.

    • Review and examine your slide sections for visible agglutinations. Compare your result with your ABO Blood System Chart. What is your blood type?

IV. Clinical Applications: Diseases of Blood

A.

TABLE 15-2 Clinical Applications on Blood Conditions

DISEASE/CONDITION	DEFINITION/FEATURES
ANEMIA	Inadequate or lack of O_2 carrying capacity by blood to tissues.
▪ IRON DEFICIENCY	Anemia due to nutritional deficiency of iron (Fe), required for RBC synthesis. Most common anemia worldwide.
▪ VITAMIN B12 DEFICIENCY	Anemia due to nutritional deficiency of vitamin B12, required for RBC synthesis. Also called **pernicious anemia**. Intrinsic factor (produced by stomach) is required for B12 absorption in the terminal ileum of GI.
▪ SICKLE CELL	Inherited. Defective hemoglobin makes the RBC less flexible and predisposed to "sickling" and unable to travel through narrowed blood vessels leading to blockage and lack of O_2 (ischemia) and subsequent tissue infarction.
▪ THALASSEMIA	Inherited. Defective or absent hemoglobin chains lead to ischemia and tissue infarction.
CYTOPENIAS	Decrease or lack of blood cells.
▪ THROMBOCYTOPENIA	Decrease or lack of platelet production. Risk of bleeding or increase in inability to clot
▪ NEUTROPENIA	Decrease or lack of leukocytes (WBCs).
CYTOSIS	Elevated blood elements. May predispose to thrombosis.
▪ ERYTHROCYTOSIS	Elevated red blood cells. **Polycythemia:** an abnormally high RBC, which may be reactive to dehydration and hypoxia, or due to bone marrow disorder of unknown etiology (**Polycythemia vera**). May predispose to thrombosis.
▪ LEUKOCYTOSIS	Elevated leukocytes (WBCs). May be due to infection, fever, stress, and exercise. The accompanying **neutrophilia** is elevated neutrophil specific.
▪ THROMBOCYTOSIS	Elevated thrombocytes (platelets). May predispose to thrombosis.
▪ INFECTIOUS MONONUCLEOSIS	Elevated monocytes (monocytosis) due to Epstein–Barr viral infection. Symptoms of fever, lethargy, and sore throat. Enlarged nodes (and spleen) may persist for 4–6 weeks. Treatment: bed rest, fluids, and analgesics.
HEMOPHILIA	X-linked inherited bleeding disorder. Absence of Clotting Factor VIII (most common) or IX leads to spontaneous bleeding. Treated with Clotting Factor transfusion.
von WILLIBRAND DISEASE	Inherited bleeding disorder. Absence of von Willibrand Clotting Factor (which is associated with Clotting Factor VIII) also leads to spontaneous bleeding despite normal platelets.
LEUKEMIA	Unknown cause. A type of cancer. Proliferation of one of the WBC element types from the stem cells in the bone marrow, producing abnormally immature cells that are nonfunctional into the blood periphery. Leukocytosis with anemia is common.
HEMATOCRIT	Number of RBCs per volume of whole blood or the percentage of RBCs in blood sample. Used to screen or treat patient for anemia.

V. Post-Lab Activity: Cardiovascular System: Blood: Identify And Label These Structures

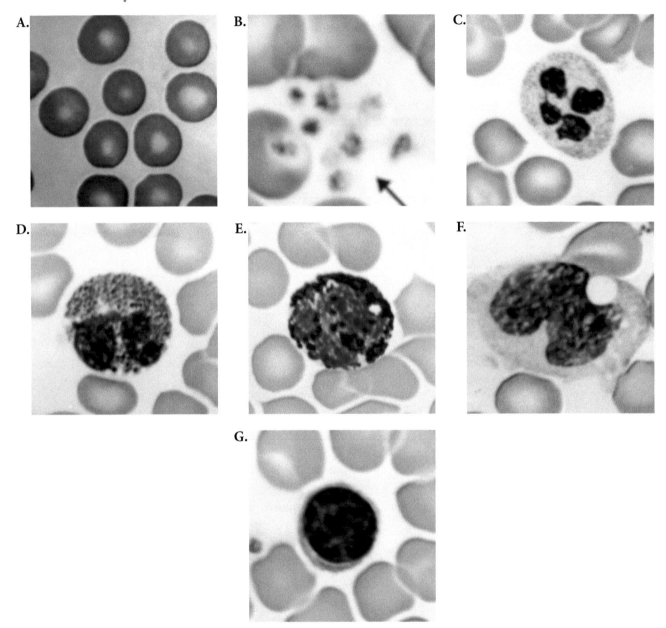

FIGURE 15-9 Identify Blood Slide A to G.

A. IDENTIFY AND LABEL BLOOD ELEMENTS ON TISSUE SLIDES:

i) **Basophil ii) Eosinophil iii) Neutrophil iv) Lymphocytes v) Monocytes vi) Platelets vii) Red blood cells viii) Sickle cell anemia ix) Whole blood**

B. **1.** Distinguish between plasma and blood.

2. Name the two most abundant white blood cell types in the blood.

3. Sketch each of the leukocytes with their characteristic features and list their functions.

4. Sketch the sickle cell slide with their characteristic feature.

C. Answer the following:
1. The major protein in the RBCs is
   A. myoglobin
   B. fibrinogen
   C. albumin
   D. hemoglobin
2. This ABO blood type is considered the universal donor:
   A. group O
   B. group A
   C. group B
   D. group AB
3. Platelets are considered fragments of these cells
   A. erythroblasts
   B. myeloblasts
   C. lymphoblasts
   D. megakaryocytes
4. This is the most abundant plasma protein
   A. lipoproteins
   B. albumins
   C. fibrinogens
   D. globulins
5. Define the major functions of the RBCs.
6. List and define the functions each of the five leukocytes.

Heart

LEARNING OUTCOMES

Upon completion of this exercise, you should be able to:

A. Describe the location and coverings of the heart in the thoracic cavity.
B. Describe the external structures of the heart.
C. Identify the major blood vessels of the heart.
D. Identify and describe the function of the main internal structures of the heart.
E. Describe the following blood flow: pulmonary, systemic, and coronary.
F. Conduction system of the heart and diagnostic use of electrocardiogram (EKG)
G. List the clinical application.

NEEDED MATERIALS

1. Human torso
2. Heart model
3. EKG strip
4. Sheep heart
5. Dissection kit with tray

Introduction

I. OVERVIEW

A. The human heart weighs approximately 350 g or the size of your fist and located in the anterior media sternum cavity (behind the sternum).
B. Two-third is located to the left of midsagittal plane.
C. Apex: Inferior aspect points toward the left hip.
D. Base: superior aspect, where major blood vessels enter and leave the heart.
E. Consider a "dual pump-in one" (right and left) but works in synchrony.

II. Lab Activity Ex: 16-1: Using the Heart Models

A.

Identify the following cardiovascular structures on the models

Heart External–Internal

- apex of heart
- pericardial cavity
- parietal pericardium
- epicardium
- myocardium
- endocardium
- atria and auricles
- ventricles
- interventricular septum
- tricuspid valve
- bicuspid/mitral valve
- semilunar valves (aortic and pulmonary)
- chordae tendineae
- papillary muscles
- superior vena cava
- inferior vena cava
- pulmonary artery
- pulmonary veins

Aorta

- ascending, arch, descending
- aortic arch
- brachiocephalic artery
- R. common carotid artery
- R. subclavian artery
- left common carotid artery
- left subclavian artery

Coronary vessels

- right coronary artery
- marginal artery

- posterior interventricular artery
- left coronary artery
- anterior interventricular artery (left anterior descending, LAD)
- circumflex artery
- coronary sinus
- great cardiac vein
- middle cardiac vein
- ligamentum arteriosum
- fossa ovale
- coronary sinus opening
- Septum: interventricular/interatria

Identify these conducting features on paper/diagram

- sinoatrial (SA) node
- atrioventricular (AV) node
- Bundle of His
- bundle branches
- Purkinje fibers
- electrocardiogram (ECG): parts
  - P wave
  - QRS complex
  - T wave
- EKG rate/rhythm calculation
- bradycardia
- tachycardia
- fibrillation (atrial/ventricular)
- ectopic beat (PVC or PAC)
- heart block: first- and second-degree AV block

A1.
TABLE 16-1 External Heart Structures

STRUCTURE	DESCRIPTION/FUNCTION
PARIETAL PERICARDIUM	Thick outer fibrous connective tissue covering the heart.
VISCERAL PERICARDIUM	Thin inner membrane clings to the heart; it is continuous with the epicardium.
AURICLES (2) RIGHT AND LEFT	External leaflets (ear-like) of atria, expand to accommodate excess fluid in the atrial.
RIGHT ATRIAL–VENTRICULAR (AV) SULCUS/GROOVE	Located between the right atria and right ventricle. Right coronary artery and Small cardiac vein travels here.
LEFT ATRIAL–VENTRICULAR (AV) SULCUS/GROOVE	Located between the left atria and left ventricle. Circumflex artery (left coronary artery branch) and Small cardiac vein travels here.
ANTERIOR INTER–VENTRICULAR SULCUS/GROOVE	Located between the right and left ventricles along interventricular septum. Left anterior descending artery (LAD) and (left coronary artery branch) and Small cardiac vein travels here.
SUPERIOR VENA CAVA	Receives deoxygenated venous blood from head-neck and upper extremities. Empties into the right atrium.
INFERIOR VENA CAVA	Receives deoxygenated venous blood from abdomen and lower extremities. Empties into the right atrium.
AORTA	Receives oxygenated blood from left ventricle and conveys to the rest of the blood.
ASCENDING AORTA	First (rising) segment of the aorta. The roots of both the right and left coronary arteries are here.
AORTIC ARCH	Second segment of the aorta. Gives rise to 3 major arterial branches (brachiocephalic, left common carotid, and subclavian arteries).
LIGAMENTUM ARTERIOSUS	Whitish fibrous ligament between pulmonary trunk and arch of aorta. A remnant of fetal circulation. During intrauterine life was an open tube (ductus arteriosus) that bypasses the non-functioning lung.
BRACHIOCEPHALIC TRUNK (ARTERY)	The first major artery of the arch of aorta. Immediately divides into 2: right common carotid artery and right subclavian arteries. Supply the right side head-neck and right upper extremity.
LEFT COMMON CAROTID ARTERY	The second major artery off the arch of aorta. Will later divide into 2: left internal and external carotid arteries. Supply the left side head-neck.
LEFT SUBCLAVIAN ARTERY	The third major artery of the arch of aorta. Supply the left upper extremity.
DESCENDING AORTA	Descends into thorax, becomes the thoracic and abdominal aorta.
PULMONARY TRUNK (ARTERY)	Anterior lateral to the aorta. Receives deoxygenated blood from right ventricle and delivers it into the lungs. Only artery in the body that carries deoxygenated blood.
PULMONARY VEINS (R AND L)	Receives oxygenated blood from lungs and delivers it into the left atrium. Only veins in the body that carries oxygenated blood.
POSTERIOR INTER–VENTRICULAR SULCUS/GROOVE	Posterior interventricular artery and middle cardiac vein travel in this.
CORONARY SULCUS	A venous bulge on the posterior wall. All cardiac veins drain into this. Then it empties into right atrium medial wall (coronary sinus opening).

B.

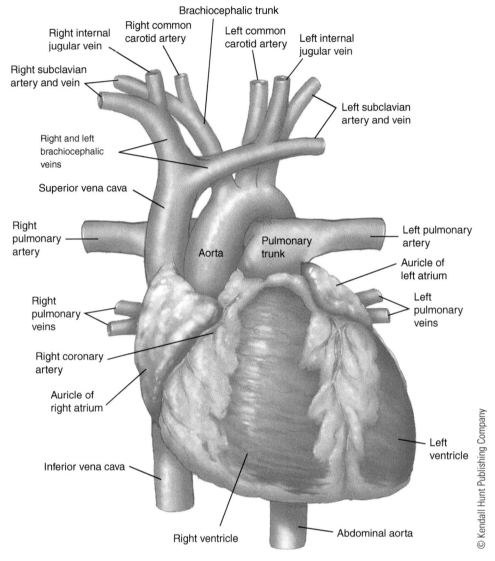

Brachiocephalic trunk

Right common carotid artery

Left common carotid artery

Right internal jugular vein

Left internal jugular vein

Right subclavian artery and vein

Left subclavian artery and vein

Right and left brachiocephalic veins

Superior vena cava

Right pulmonary artery

Aorta

Pulmonary trunk

Left pulmonary artery

Auricle of left atrium

Right pulmonary veins

Left pulmonary veins

Right coronary artery

Auricle of right atrium

Left ventricle

Inferior vena cava

Right ventricle

Abdominal aorta

© Kendall Hunt Publishing Company

FIGURE 16-1 Heart- Anterior View

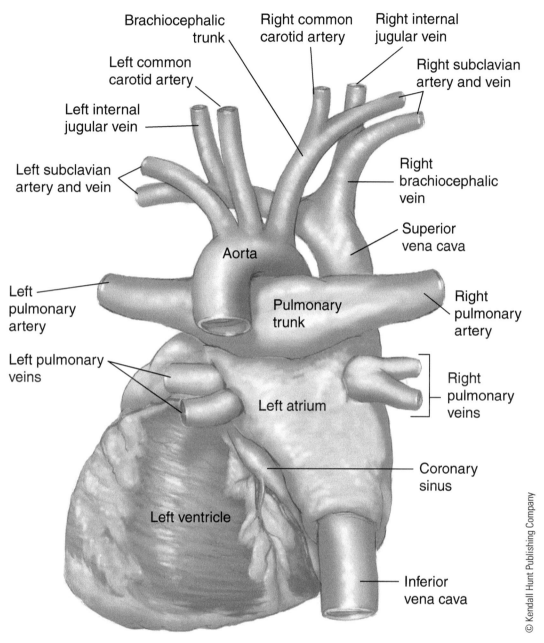

Brachiocephalic trunk

Right common carotid artery

Right internal jugular vein

Left common carotid artery

Right subclavian artery and vein

Left internal jugular vein

Left subclavian artery and vein

Right brachiocephalic vein

Aorta

Superior vena cava

Left pulmonary artery

Pulmonary trunk

Right pulmonary artery

Left pulmonary veins

Right pulmonary veins

Left atrium

Coronary sinus

Left ventricle

Inferior vena cava

© Kendall Hunt Publishing Company

FIGURE 16-2 Heart- Posterior View

III. Internal Heart Structures

A.

TABLE 16-2 Internal Heart Structures

STRUCTURE	DESCRIPTION/FUNCTION
EPICARDIUM	Outermost layer, and is continuous with the visceral pericardium.
MYOCARDIUM	Middle layer muscular wall of the heart, responsible for contractility.
ENDOCARDIUM	Inner lining (simple squamous epithelium) of the heart in contact with blood.
RIGHT ATRIUM	Receives deoxygenated blood from systemic circulation. All venous blood returns here EXCEPT pulmonary veins (which return to left atrium). Empties into LV during diastolic filling.
INTER ATRIAL SEPTUM	Separates the 2 atria cavities.
FOSSA OVALES	Indent located on the medial wall of right atrium. A remnant of fetal circulation, previously foramen ovales: shunts blood from right atria into left atria. Closes after first breath in the newborn.
CORONARY SULCUS OPENING	Opening of the coronary sinus (venous) as it empties into right atrium medial wall.
LEFT ATRIUM	Receives oxygenated blood via pulmonary veins from lungs only.
RIGHT ATRIA-VENTRICULAR (AV) VALVES (TRICUSPID)	An inlet valve with 3 leaflets. Located between RA and RV. Opens during ventricular diastole to allow venous blood to fill the right ventricle from right atrial.
LEFT ATRIA-VENTRICULAR (AV) VALVES (BICUSPID)	An inlet valve with 2 leaflets. Also called MITRAL VALVE. Located between LA and LV. Opens during ventricular diastole to allow venous blood to fill the left ventricle from left atrial.
PULMONARY SEMI-LUNA VALVE	An outlet valve. Leads away from RV. Opens during ventricular systole to allow deoxygenated blood to leave from the right ventricle into the lungs.
AORTIC SEMI-LUNA VALVE	An outlet valve. Leads away from LV. Opens during ventricular systole to allow oxygenated blood to leave from the left ventricle into systemic circulation.
CHORDAE TENDINAE	Chord-like tendons, holds the AV valves and tethered to the papillary muscles inside the ventricular cavities.
PAPILLARY MUSCLES	Pillar-like muscle structures; are part of the ventricular inner wall. The chordae tendineae attach the AV valves (tricuspid and mitral valves) to the papillary muscles.
TRABECULAE CARNAE	Maze-like network of inner ventricular muscle projections.
RIGHT VENTRICLE	Has thinner wall than LV. Receives venous (deoxygenated blood) from RA. Then dumps it into the lungs via pulmonary trunk (artery).
LEFT VENTRICLE	Thicker (muscular) wall than the RV. Receives oxygenated blood from LA. Then dumps it into the systemic circulation via aorta (artery).
INTERVENTRICULAR SEPTUM	Thick muscular structure separates the LV and RV.
SUPERIOR VENA CAVA OPENING	Found in the roof of the right atrium.
INFERIOR VENA CAVA OPENING	Found on the inferior aspect of the right atrium.

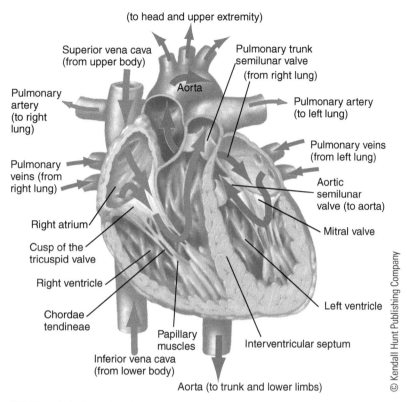

(to head and upper extremity)

Superior vena cava
(from upper body)

Pulmonary trunk
semilunar valve
(from right lung)

Aorta

Pulmonary
artery
(to right
lung)

Pulmonary artery
(to left lung)

Pulmonary veins
(from left lung)

Pulmonary
veins (from
right lung)

Aortic
semilunar
valve (to aorta)

Right atrium

Mitral valve

Cusp of the
tricuspid valve

Right ventricle

Left ventricle

Chordae
tendineae

Papillary
muscles

Interventricular septum

Inferior vena cava
(from lower body)

Aorta (to trunk and lower limbs)

© Kendall Hunt Publishing Company

FIGURE 16-3 Heart Interior

IIIA. Lab Activity 16-2 Dissection of the Sheep Heart

A. Sheep Heart Dissection Instruction:

1. Open your package of preserved sheep heart. Rinse off in water thoroughly to remove the preservative as possible. Also run water into the larger blood vessels to force any blood clots out of the heart chambers.

2. Place the heart on a dissecting tray with its ventral surface. Identify the anterior surface and posterior structures listed.

3. Open and expose the interior heart, as follows:
   - Insert a blade of a sharp scalpel or knife and cut from the apex upwards into two halves toward the base where the great vessels are located.

4. Locate and identify the listed structures.

B. Sheep Heart Dissection: Locate and Identify the following structures:

**Ventral View
(with Coronary Arteries)**
1. Anterior interventricular artery
2. Aorta
3. Brachiocephalic artery
4. Cardiac veins
5. Circumflex artery
6. Coronary sinus
7. Inferior vena cava
8. Left atrium
9. Left common carotid artery
10. Left coronary artery

**Dorsal View
(with Cardiac Veins)**
11. Left pulmonary artery
12. Left pulmonary vein
13. Left subclavian artery
14. Left ventricle
15. Marginal artery
16. Posterior interventricular artery
17. Right atrium
18. Right coronary artery
19. Right pulmonary vein
20. Right ventricle
21. Superior vena cava

Internal View
22. Right atrium
23. Left atrium
24. Tricuspid valve
25. Bicuspid (Mitra) valve
26. Fossa ovale
27. Coronary sinus opening
28. Chordae tendineae
29. Papillary muscles
30. Trabeculae carnae
31. Interventricular septum
32. Interatria septum
33. Pulmonary valve
34. Aortic valve

IV. Lab Activity 16-3 Pulmonary Circulation

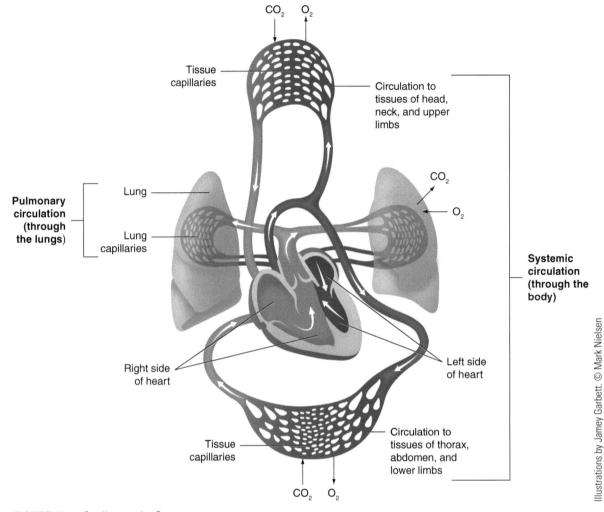

FIGURE 16-4 Cardiovascular System

Illustrations by Jamey Garbett. © Mark Nielsen

A. We will trace a drop of blood (deoxygenated) returning to right atrium from any organ(s) through the heart, then to and from the lungs:

B. RA (DEOXYGENATED BLOOD) ⟶ TRICUSPID VALVE ⟶ RV ⟶ PULMONARY TRUNK/VALVE ⟶ LUNGS (OXYGENATED BLOOD) ⟶ PULMONARY VEINS ⟶ LA

V. Lab Activity 16-4: Systemic Circulation

A. We will trace a drop of blood (oxygenated) retuned to LA from the lungs through organ systems and back to the right side of the heart.

B. LA (OXYGENATED BLOOD) ⟶ BICUSPID/MITRAL VALVE ⟶ LV ⟶ AORTIC VALVE/AORTA ⟶ MAJOR ARTERIES ⟶ CAPILLARIES ⟶ ORGANS ⟶ VEINS (DEOXYGENATED BLOOD) ⟶ MAJOR VEINS (IVC/SVC) ⟶ RA

C. NOTE: All blood returns to the heart:

1. Via veins and

2. Majority return into RA and are DEOXYGENATED BLOOD

3. EXCEPT: Blood returning from lung:

   ■ Returns into LA

   ■ Via pulmonary veins which carry oxygenated blood

VI. Great Heart Vessels

TABLE 16-3 Major Heart Blood Vessels

STRUCTURE	DESCRIPTION/FUNCTION
SUPERIOR VENA CAVA	Receives deoxygenated venous blood from head-neck and upper extremities. Empties into the right atrium.
INFERIOR VENA CAVA	Receives deoxygenated venous blood from abdomen and lower extremities. Empties into the right atrium.
AORTA	Receives oxygenated blood from left ventricle and conveys to the rest of the blood.
ASCENDING AORTA	1st (rising) segment of the aorta. The roots of both the right and left coronary arteries are here.
AORTIC ARCH	2nd segment of the aorta. Gives rise to the 3 major arterial branches (brachiocephalic, left common carotid, & subclavian arteries).
BRACHIOCEPHALIC TRUNK (ARTERY)	The 1st major artery of the arch of aorta. Immediately divides into 2: right common carotid artery & right subclavian arteries. Supply the right side head-neck & right upper extremity.
LEFT COMMON CAROTID ARTERY	The 2nd major artery of the arch of aorta. Will later divide into 2: Left internal & external carotid arteries. Supply the left side head-neck.
LEFT SUBCLAVIAN ARTERY	The 3rd major artery of the arch of aorta. Supply the left upper extremity.
DESCENDING AORTA	Descends into thorax, becomes the thoracic & abdominal aorta.
PULMONARY TRUNK (ARTERY)	Anterior lateral to the aorta. Receives deoxygenated blood from right ventricle and delivers it into the lungs. Only artery in the body that carries deoxygenated blood.
PULMONARY VEINS (R & L)	Receives oxygenated blood from lungs and delivers it into the left atrium. Only veins in the body that carries oxygenated blood.
RIGHT COMMON CAROTID ARTERY	Branch off the brachiocephalic trunk (1 of 2 branches). Will later divide into 2: right internal & external carotid arteries. Supply the right side head-neck.
RIGHT SUBCLAVIAN ARTERY	Branch off the brachiocephalic trunk (2 of 2 branches). Supply the right upper extremity.
CORONARY SULCUS	A venous bulge on the posterior wall. All cardiac veins drain into this. Then it empties into right atrium medial wall (coronary sinus opening).

A. Definitions:
   i. Arteries: All Carry Blood Away From The Heart And Are Oxygenated Blood
   ii. Except: Pulmonary Artery (Trunk), Carries Deoxygenated Blood Away From Heart To The Lungs.
   iii. Veins: All Carry Blood To The Heart And Are Deoxygenated Blood.
   iv. Except: Pulmonary Veins, Which Carry Oxygenated Blood Toward The Heart (La) From Lungs.

VII. Coronary Blood Flow/Circulation

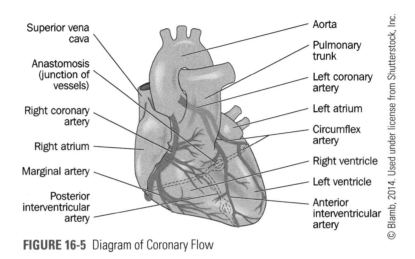

Superior vena cava

Anastomosis (junction of vessels)

Right coronary artery

Right atrium

Marginal artery

Posterior interventricular artery

Aorta

Pulmonary trunk

Left coronary artery

Left atrium

Circumflex artery

Right ventricle

Left ventricle

Anterior interventricular artery

© Blamb, 2014. Used under license from Shutterstock, Inc.

FIGURE 16-5 Diagram of Coronary Flow

A. Oxygenation (arterial) to the myocardium is during ventricular DIASTOLE from the backflow of blood back into the root of the aorta and into the coronary arteries.

TABLE 16-4 Cell Structure and Function

STRUCTURE	DESCRIPTION/FUNCTION
RIGHT CORONARY ARTERY (RCA)	Originates from the root of the aorta behind the pulmonary trunk. Travels in the right AV sulcus, supplies right atrium and right ventricle. And gives rise to right marginal artery. RCA continues in the posterior interventricular sulcus and anastomoses with the circumflex branch (of LCA).
RIGHT MARGINAL ARTERY	A branch of the right coronary artery; descends toward the apex; supplies blood to the right lateral side of the heart.
LEFT CORONARY ARTERY (LCA)	Aka "left main." Originates from the root of the aorta behind the pulmonary trunk, gives rise to circumflex artery and left anterior descending (LAD).
LEFT CIRCUMFLEX ARTERY	First major branch of the LCA. Travels laterally around the left side of the heart in the left AV sulcus to supply blood to the left atrium and posterior side of the left ventricle. Anastomoses with the RCA.
ANTERIOR (INTERVENTRICULAR) ARTERY	Aka "left anterior descending (LAD) artery." Second major branch of the LCA. Travels in anterior interventricular sulcus and supplies the left auricle, left ventricle, interventricular septum, and much of the anterior heart.
LEFT MARGINAL ARTERY	A branch of the circumflex artery supplies arterial blood to the left lateral side of the heart.
POST-INTERVENTRICULAR ARTERY	Travels in the posterior interventricular sulcus, toward the apex. Formed by the anastomoses (junction) of right coronary artery, LAD, and the circumflex arteries. Supplies the posterior, middle, and right sides of the myocardium.
GREAT CARDIAC VEIN	Travels with the anterior interventricular artery (LAD); drains blood from the anterior surface of the heart; travels superiorly then laterally around the heart; empties into the coronary sinus.
SMALL CARDIAC VEIN	Drains the left right lateral side of the heart; empties into the coronary sinus.
ANTERIOR CARDIAC VEIN	Primarily drains the anterior right lateral side of the heart; empties directly into the right atrium.

STRUCTURE	DESCRIPTION/FUNCTION
MIDDLE CARDIAC VEIN	Travels with the posterior interventricular artery; drains blood from the posterior surface of the heart; empties into the coronary sinus.
POSTERIOR CARDIAC VEIN	Drains the posterior and left lateral side before emptying into the coronary sinus.
CORONARY SINUS	A venous bulge on the posterior heart wall. All cardiac veins drain into this. Then it empties into right atrium medial wall (as coronary sinus opening).

VIII. Lab Activity 16-5 Conducting System of the Heart

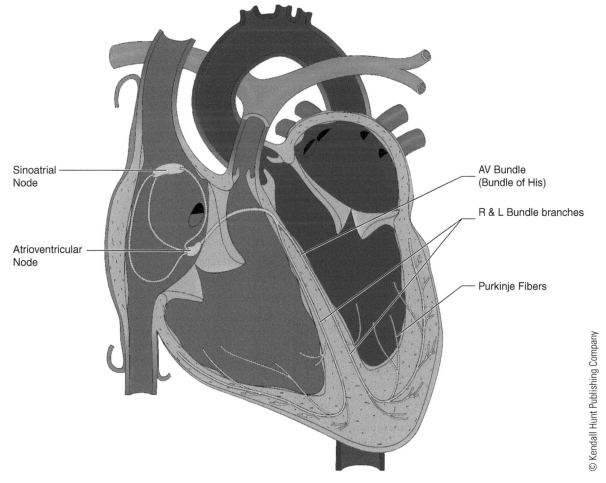

Sinoatrial Node

Atrioventricular Node

AV Bundle (Bundle of His)

R & L Bundle branches

Purkinje Fibers

© Kendall Hunt Publishing Company

FIGURE 16-6

A. The conducting system of the heart is made up of modified cardiac muscle. The SA node acts as the "pacemaker," setting the pace for heart rate (60–100/minute). Other sections (below the SA node to the ventricles) are capable of spontaneous depolarization but at a much slower pace (below 60).

B. Action potential traveling in the myocardium:

SA NODE ⟶ RA ⟶ LA ⟶ AV NODE ⟶ AV BUNDLE (HIS) ⟶ R & L BUNDLE BRANCHES ⟶ PURKINJE FIBERS

TABLE 16-5 Heart Conducting System

STRUCTURE	DESCRIPTION AND FUNCTION
SINOATRIAL NODE (PACE-MAKER)	Located in the sulcus terminalis close to the opening of the superior vena cava. It initiates heartbeat; blood supply is often by the right coronary artery. Spontaneously depolarizes sending impulses to both atria and AV node below.
ATRIOVENTRICULAR NODE (AV NODE)	Located in the lower part of the atrial septum (and close to the AV junction). Receives stimulus from the SA node. Its blood supply is by the right coronary artery.
ATRIOVENTRICULAR BUNDLE (BUNDLE OF HIS)	It is continuous with the AV node above and the bundle branches below. Receives stimulus from the AV node, sends impulses to bundle branches.
BUNDLE BRANCHES (R&L)	The AV bundle divides into right bundle branches traveling in the right ventricular wall and the left bundle branches traveling in the left ventricular wall. Both terminate as Purkinje fibers or plexus. The blood supply is often by the left coronary artery.
PURKINJE PLEXUS	Terminal fibers of the conducting system within the walls of the ventricles.

IX. Lab Activity 16-6 Electrocardiogram (EKG); Identify EKG Parts and Abnormal EKG Strips

A. EKG deflections: are representations of heart *excitation* (or electrical activity) and NOT *contraction/relaxation* (or muscular activity).

B. May see a positive or negative wave deflection from baseline.

C. The cotraction/relaxation: of cardiac muscle follows the deflections (excitations) and are represented in the EKG segments. (Ex ST-segment is ventricular contraction)

C.

ECG and electrical activity of the myocardium

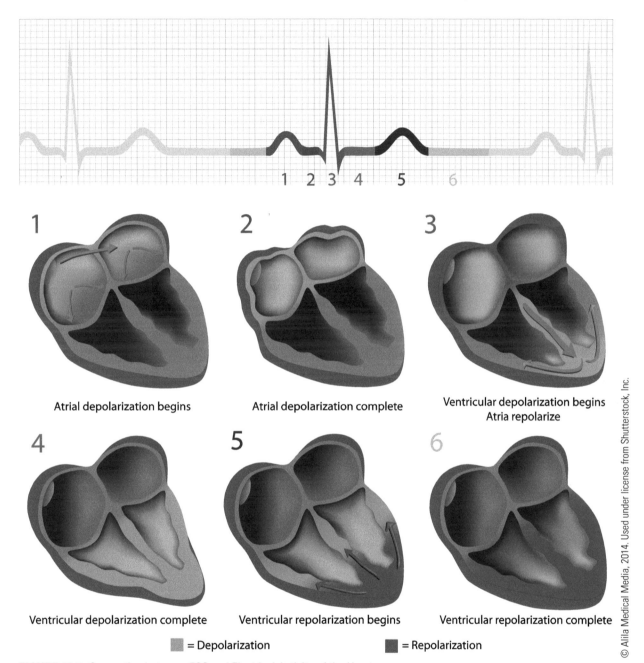

| 1 | 2 | 3 | 4 | 5 | 6 |

1
Atrial depolarization begins

2
Atrial depolarization complete

3
Ventricular depolarization begins
Atria repolarize

4
Ventricular depolarization complete

5
Ventricular repolarization begins

6
Ventricular repolarization complete

 = Depolarization   = Repolarization

FIGURE 16-7 Connection between ECG and Electrical Activity of the Heart

D.

TABLE 16-6 **EKG**

WAVE/EVENT	DESCRIPTION/REPRESENTATION
P WAVE	First wave, denotes atrial excitation/depolarization (over both atria).
PQ SEGMENT	Represents: atrial contraction (follows atrial depolarization) and continued traveling of the depolarization toward the ventricles. Time interval from atrial depolarization to ventricular depolarization (less than 0.2 second).
QRS COMPLEX	Second wave represents ventricle depolarization (over both).
ST SEGMENT	Denotes ventricular contraction.
T WAVE	Final wave: ventricular repolarization. NOTE: Atrial repolarization wave is NOT seen because it happened during ventricular depolarization and buried in the QRS complex.
QT INTERVAL	Depends on heart rate. With increased heart rate, QT interval decreases.

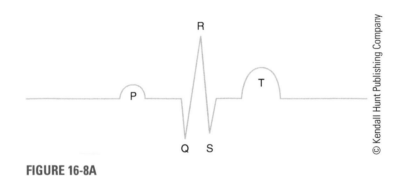

© Kendall Hunt Publishing Company

FIGURE 16-8A

E.

FIG 16-8B **METHODS OF DETERMINING EKG RATE & RYTHYM**

- All assumes a recording speed of 25mm/sec on the EKG paper/machine.

METHOD I: "Small Boxes/R-R Interval Count"

- Count the number of small boxes for a typical R-R Interval.
- Divide 1500 by that number to determine approximate heart rate.
- Ex: In Fig 1, the R-R interval is 21.5
  - Heart Rate = 1500/21.5 = 69.8 beats/min

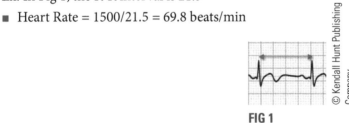

© Kendall Hunt Publishing Company

FIG 1

METHOD II: "QRS Interval Count"

- Count the number of QRS complexes over a 6 second interval
- Multiply that number by 10, to determine approximate heart rate

- Ex: In Fig 2: From Starting point 1 to End point 7, there are 6 second intervals OR
  - 7 x 10 = 70 beats/min

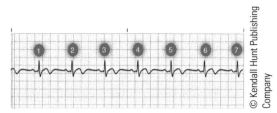

FIG 2

METHOD III: "Large Square Box Count"
- Count the number of large square boxes (red boxes plus any extra smaller boxes in Fig 2 above)
- Divide 300 by that number
- Ex: 300/4.4 = 68 beats/min

METHOD IV: "Count-Off" Method
- Ideal for regular heart rates
- Use this sequence: 300-150-100-75-60-50-43-37
- Count from the first QRS complex, the first bold line is 300, then the next bold line is 150, and so on.
- Stop the sequence count at the next QRS complex
- If the second QRS is in between 2 bold lines, take the mean of the 2 numbers from the sequence.
  - Ex: The second QRS here (Fig 3) is between "count-off" 75 and 60
  - Mean of 135 = 68 beats/min

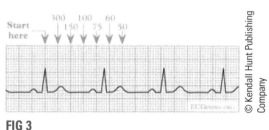

FIG 3

RYTHYM DETERMINATION

A. SINUS RYTHYM: See Fig 3
- P wave always precede the QRS complex
- Ex: Fig 3 above is Sinus Rhythm but specifically:
  - Normal Rate (60–100) and Sinus Rhythm
  - If Rate is > 100, then it's Sinus Tachycardia
  - If Rate is < 60, then it's Sinus Bradycardia

B. JUNCTIONAL (NODAL) RYTHYM: See Fig 4
- No P wave preceding the normal QRQ complex, indicating the conduction to the ventricle is not from the Sinus Node/Atrial but below it
  - AV Node or AV Bundle conduction
- Rate is usually 40–60

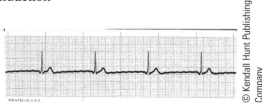

FIG 4 Junctional Rythm

C. VENTRICULAR RYTHYM: See Fig 5

- No P waves
- Widened (abnormal) QRS complexes
- Rate is variable may be:
    - Occasional Premature Ventricular Contractions (PVC's) within a Normal EKG
    - Ventricular tachycardia: Rate > 100 with no P waves, saw tooth-like waves
    - Ventricular Fibrillation: coarse or fine waves with no distinct P or QRS waves
        - Chaotic electrical activity (heart quivering like jello)
        - Results in Death in minutes.
        - Treatment: Defibrillation

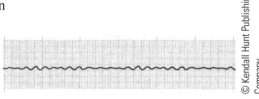

© Kendall Hunt Publishing Company

FIG 5 Ventricular Fibrillation

D. MYOCARDIAL INFARCTION vs ISCHEMIA: See Fig 6

- Marked ST Elevation in multiple EKG Leads
    - As compared to Ischemia with marked ST Depression

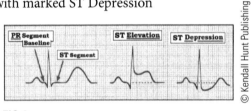

© Kendall Hunt Publishing Company

FIG 6

F.

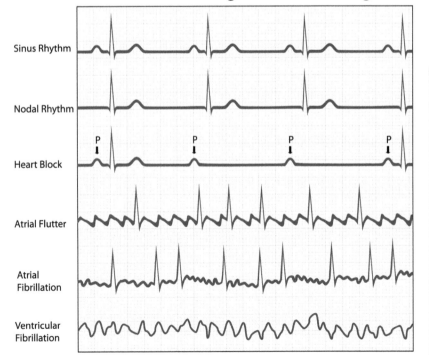

Normal and Pathological Electrocardiograms

1. Normal Sinus Rhythm and rate. P wave always before QRS Rate < 100

2. Nodal Rhythm and bradycardia. No P wave before QRS. Depolarization started at AV Node Rate < 60

3. Not all P waves conduct through to the ventricle (skipping).

4. "Saw-tooth" atrial waves some conducting others not through to ventricles, with an irregular Rate > 100

5. Chaotic atria conduction, atria waves are finer (and more dangerous) than in Atrial flutter.

6. Chaotic ventricular conduction, ventricular waves are finer (and more dangerous) than in ventricular flutter (Not shown). Immediate defibrillation or death.

© Alila Medical Media, 2014. Used under license from Shutterstock, Inc.

FIGURE 16-9 Identify Abnormal EKG strips

X. Valvular Mechanics and Heart Sounds

A. A complete cardiac cycle (1 systole and 1 diastole) involves one atria contraction and one ventricular relaxation **PLUS** one atria relaxation and one ventricular contraction. Heart valves open and close during these phases.

B. Both heart sounds S1 and S2 ("Lubb-Dubb") are due to valve closures, whereas S3 and S4 are murmurs (turbulent flow across a valve [closed, partially closed, or opened])

C.

TABLE 16-7 Valvular Mechanics-Heart Sounds

STRUCTURE/EVENT	DESCRIPTION/FUNCTION
RIGHT ATRIA-VENTRICULAR (AV) VALVES (TRICUSPID)	An inlet valve with 3 leaflets. Located between RA and RV. Opens during ventricular diastole to allow venous blood to fill the right ventricle from right atrial.
LEFT ATRIA-VENTRICULAR (AV) VALVES (BICUSPID)	An inlet valve with 2 leaflets. Also called MITRAL VALVE. Located between LA and LV. Opens during ventricular diastole to allow venous blood to fill the left ventricle from left atrial.
PULMONARY SEMI-LUNA VALVE	An outlet valve. Leads away from RV. Opens during ventricular systole to allow deoxygenated blood to leave from the right ventricle into the lungs.
AORTIC SEMI-LUNA VALVE	An outlet valve. Leads away from LV. Opens during ventricular systole to allow oxygenated blood to leave from the left ventricle into systemic circulation.
HEART SOUND S1 ("LUBB") IN LUBB-DUBB	Both S1 and S2 are due to valve CLOSURES. S1 is (low pitch, long duration sound) due to closure of AV valves at the end of ventricular diastolic filling (due to rising pressure in the ventricles) and just prior to the beginning of ventricular contraction (systole/ejection).
HEART SOUND S2 ("DUB") IN LUB-DUB	Both S1 and S2 are due to valve CLOSURES. S2 is (high pitched, sharp, short duration sound) due to closure of SL valves at the end of ventricular systole (contraction) and just prior to the beginning of ventricular relaxation (diastole/filling). Backflow of blood in the SL valves of aorta and pulmonary closes these valves resulting in S2 sound.
HEART SOUND S3	Considered a systolic murmur, heard after S1. Location of where heard and its radiation on the chest would determine which valve(s) is involved. Often due to murmur (turbulence of blood flow) across a valve.
HEART SOUND S4	Considered a diastolic murmur, heard after S2. Location of where heard and its radiation on the chest would determine which valve(s) is involved. Often due to murmur (turbulence of blood flow) across a valve.

XI. Clinical Applications Heart Diseases

A.

TABLE 16-8 Clinical Applications

DISEASE	DESCRIPTION
TACHYCARDIA	Heart rate greater than 100 BPM.
BRADYCARDIA	Heart rate less than 60 BPM.
ANGINA PECTORIS	Chest pain secondary to coronary artery narrowing (arteriosclerosis/vascular spasm) especially at rest.
ACUTE MYOCARDIAC INFARCTION (AMI)	Sudden myocardial tissue death usually due to a clot/thrombus in the coronary artery.
ACUTE CORONARY SYNDROME	Combined term used for an AMI or unstable angina.
VALVULAR STENOSIS	Denotes narrowing of the valve opening, commonly in the aortic or pulmonary valve.
VALVULAR REGURGITATION	Denotes backflow (leaking) of blood through a closed valve, may be any of the 4 heart valves: aortic/bicuspid/tricuspid regurgitation.
CORONARY ARTERIAL DISEASE	Narrowing of the coronary vessels resulting in lack of blood supply to the myocardium. May be due to arteriosclerosis (hardening of artery) and or atherosclerosis (plaque narrowing). Both typically occur together.
MITRAL VALVE PROLAPSE	A type of regurgitation. Backflow (leaking) of blood through the closed mitral valve back into the left atrium during ventricular systole. Continued backflow in the left atrium would eventually flood the lungs, resulting in pulmonary edema.
PERICARDITIS	Inflammation of the pericardium, very painful.
MYOCARDITIS	Inflammation of the myocardium.

XII. Pre-Lab Activity: Heart

Fill in the blanks

1. The layer of the pericardial membrane that lines the cavity is called the _____.

2. List the three layers of the heart from deep to superficial:

   i. _____

   ii. _____

   iii. _____

3. The _____ side of the heart controls the flow of blood to the tissues.

4. The texture lining the atria of the heart is known as _____.

XIII. Post-Lab Activity: Heart

A. LABEL THESE STRUCTURES

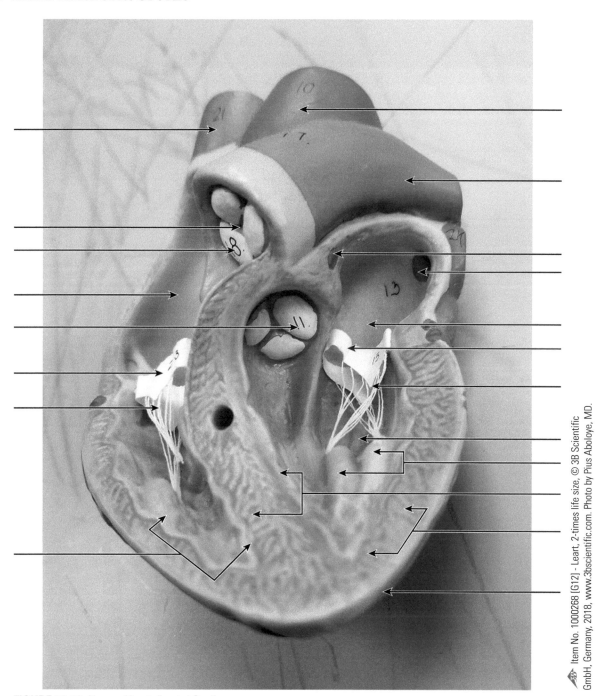

FIGURE 16-10 Human Heart, Frontal Section

Item No. 1000268 [G12] - Leart, 2-times life size, © 3B Scientific GmbH, Germany, 2018, www.3bscientific.com. Photo by Pius Aboloye, MD.

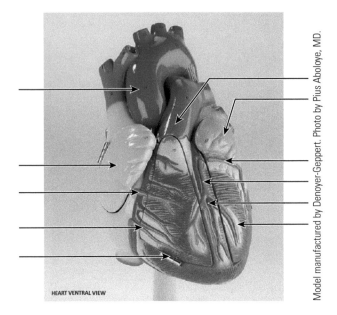

HEART VENTRAL VIEW

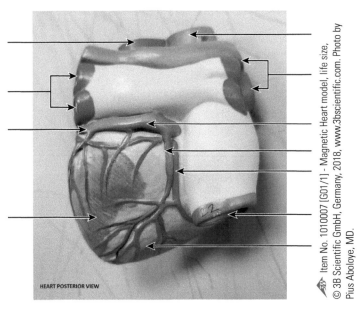

HEART POSTERIOR VIEW

FIGURE 16-11 Human Heart, Ventral and Posterior View

B.

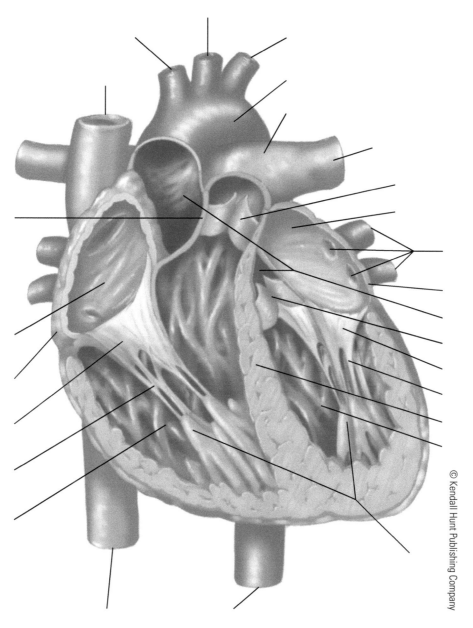

FIGURE 16-12 Diagram of the Heart (Internal)

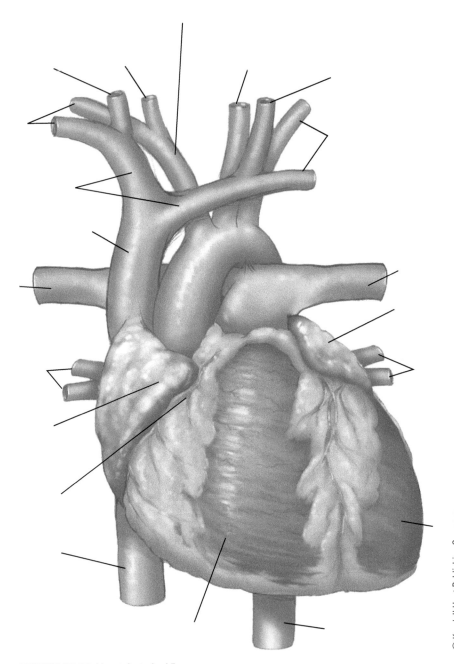

FIGURE 16-13 Heart-Anterior View

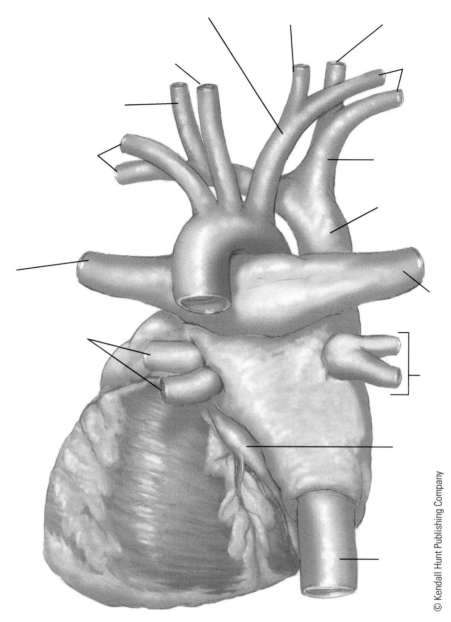

FIGURE 16-14 Heart-Posterior View

Heart Practice Quiz

1. All of the following protect the heart laterally EXCEPT:
   A. Ribs
   B. Sternum
   C. Intercostal muscles
   D. Lungs
   E. Pericardium

2. The pericardium blends: (Choose all that apply.)
   A. Into the diaphragm inferiorly
   B. Into the myocardium
   C. Into the endocardium
   D. Into the great vessels coming off the heart superiorly
   E. All of the above

3. The apex of the heart points:
   A. Superiorly and to the right
   B. Superiorly and to the left
   C. Laterally and to the left
   D. Laterally and to the right
   E. Inferiorly and to the left

4. All of the following structures contain musculi pectinati EXCEPT:
   A. Right atrium
   B. Left atrium
   C. Right auricle
   D. Left auricle

5. Choose the following that have 3 cusps: (Choose all that apply.)
   A. Right atrioventricular valve
   B. Left atrioventricular valve
   C. Pulmonary semilunar valve
   D. Aortic semilunar valve
   E. Pulmonary trunk

6. The pulmonary semilunar valve opens when:
   A. Flow is retrograde
   B. Blood moves from the left ventricle into the pulmonary trunk
   C. Blood moves from the right ventricle to the aorta
   D. When the aortic semilunar valve closes
   E. None of the above

7. All of the following are openings of the right atrium EXCEPT: (Choose all that apply.)
   A. Coronary sinus
   B. Superior vena cava
   C. Inferior vena cava
   D. Left atrioventricular valve
   E. 4 pulmonary veins

8. Heart disease: (Choose all that apply.)

   A. Is a minor problem in that United States

   B. Accounts for about 29% of all death in the United States

   C. Can lead to heart attack, which can lead to cardiac arrest

   D. Is a condition is which hardening of the arteries occurs in the arteries that supply the arms and legs

   E. In most cases is harmless

9. All of the following are false EXCEPT (Choose all that apply):

   A. Cardiac arrest cannot result in death

   B. Heart failure is when the heart cannot pump blood the way it should

   C. The heart muscles may not receive enough oxygen and begin to die during a heart attack

   D. CHD involves venosclerosis

   E. All of the above are true

10. All of the following are true regarding mitral valve prolapse EXCEPT:

   A. In most cases it is harmless

   B. May need to be treated with surgery if severe

   C. Patients may not know they have the problem

   D. A symptom may be numbness

   E. May become severe mitral regurgitation

11. Atherosclerosis is seen in all of the following EXCEPT:

   A. Heart disease

   B. CHD

   C. PAD

   D. All of the above including atherosclerosis

12. Cardiomyopathy can be caused by all of the following EXCEPT:

   A. Prior heart attacks

   B. Multiple heart defects

   C. Viral infection

   D. Bacterial infections

13. Symptoms and sign of PAD include: (Choose all that apply.)

   A. Numbness

   B. Chest pain

   C. Swelling of chest

   D. Weak pulse in feet

   E. Softening of artery walls

14. Arteriosclerosis:

   A. Is a type of atherosclerosis

   B. Cam cause blood to leak backward

   C. Is when the aorta stretches and dilates

   D. Includes irregular heartbeats

   E. None of the above

B. Answer the following questions:

1. The visceral pericardium is continuous with this layer

    A. parietal pericardium

    B. epicardium

    C. endocardium

    D. myocardium

2. The right ventricle receives blood from the

    A. systemic circuit

    B. lungs

    C. left atrium

    D. right atrium

3. The QRS wave on an EKG strip represents

    A. ventricular depolarization

    B. atrial repolarization

    C. ventricular repolarization

    D. atrial depolarization

4. The ST wave on an EKG strip represents

    A. ventricular depolarization

    B. atrial repolarization

    C. ventricular repolarization

    D. ventricular contraction

5. The difference between the systolic and diastolic pressures is referred to as

    A. pulse pressure

    B. circulatory pressure

    C. blood pressure

    D. mean arterial pressure

6. List the diagnostic lab findings on a patient having an acute myocardial infarction.

7. Trace one drop of blood through both the pulmonary and systemic circulation.

8. Explain why is the left ventricular wall much thicker than the right ventricle.

Blood Vessels

Upon completion of this exercise, you should be able to:

A. Compare and contrast the structure of arteries and veins including the tunics.
B. List the different types of arteries and veins.
C. Correlate the anatomical structure of each type of blood vessel with its function.
D. Identify the major blood vessels (arteries and veins) of the body.
E. Describe the systemic circulation.
F. Describe special circulation: cerebral flow, hepatic portal, and fetal circulation.
G. Identify the pulse pressure areas.
H. List the clinical applications.

NEEDED MATERIALS

1. Human torso.
2. Heart model.
3. Arm and leg muscle models with blood vessels.
4. Blood vessel wall plaques.
5. Artery and vein structure stand tissue slides.

Introduction

I. OVERVIEW

A. Arteries carry blood away from the heart and most often carrying oxygenated blood to organs.
B. Veins carry blood toward the heart and most often carrying deoxygenated blood from organs to the heart.
C. Three different types of arteries (large, medium, and small capillaries), hence different functions.
D. Three different types of veins (large, medium, and small venules), hence different functions.

TABLE 17-1 Blood Vessel Types

TYPE	BLOOD VESSEL	DESCRIPTION
Arteries	Elastic arteries (conducting arteries)	Have the largest luminal diameter with an abundance of elastic fibers (e.g., aorta and pulmonary trunk).
	Muscular arteries (distributing arteries)	Delivers blood to specific body regions. Distinguished by having the thickest wall of all the blood vessels and having a distinct internal elastic membrane (e.g., brachial artery and femoral artery).
	Arterioles	Deliver blood to capillary beds. Very thin.
Capillaries	Continuous capillaries	Least permeable capillary consisting of endothelium only. Abundant in skin, skeletal muscles, and brain.
	Fenestrated capillaries	Moderately permeable capillary consisting of endothelium only. Found in digestive organs and endocrine glands.
	Sinusoids	Most permeable capillary consisting of endothelium only. Located in the liver and spleen.
Veins	Venule	Formed when capillaries unite. Smallest veins. Consists of all three tunics. Unites to form veins.
	Medium-sized veins	Formed when several venules unite. Companion to the muscular arteries. Most contain numerous *valves* that prevent blood from pooling in the limbs.
	Large veins	Largest veins in the body. Deliver blood directly to the heart.

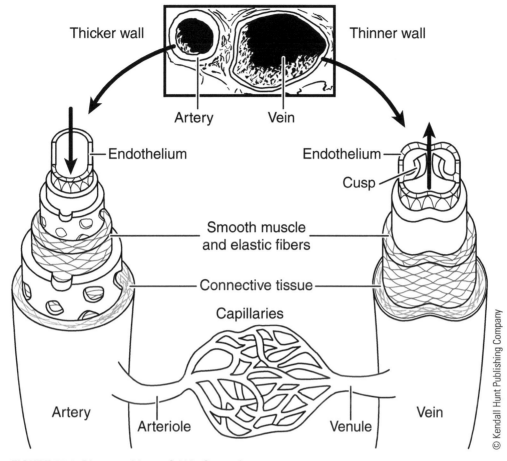

FIGURE 17-1 Diagram of Artery & Vein Comparison

© Kendall Hunt Publishing Company

TABLE 17-2 Types of Blood Vessels Compared

ARTERY	FEATURES	VEINS
Round, solid, and firm. Smaller diameter with thicker wall.	**CROSS-SECTIONAL VIEW**	Flimsy and collapsible. Larger diameter with thinner wall.
Similar.	**EXTERNAL TUNIC**	Similar.
Much thicker.	**MIDDLE TUNIC** ■ SMOOTH MUSCLE	Thinner.
Present.	■ ELASTIN FIBERS	Not present.
Rippled/rough surface second to vasoconstriction.	**INNER TUNIC**	Smoother surface.

II. Vascular Supply of the Human Body

A. MAJOR ARTERIAL SUPPLY

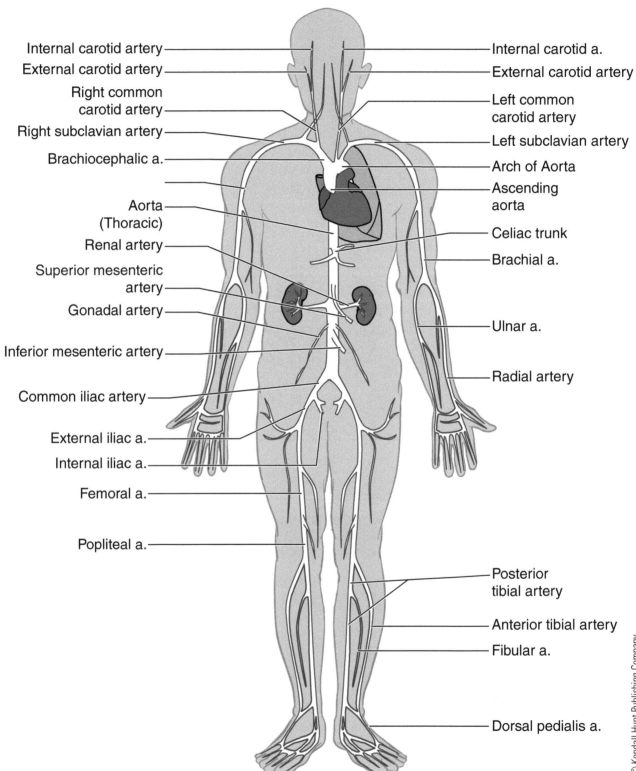

Internal carotid artery

External carotid artery

Right common carotid artery

Right subclavian artery

Brachiocephalic a.

Aorta (Thoracic)

Renal artery

Superior mesenteric artery

Gonadal artery

Inferior mesenteric artery

Common iliac artery

External iliac a.

Internal iliac a.

Femoral a.

Popliteal a.

Internal carotid a.

External carotid artery

Left common carotid artery

Left subclavian artery

Arch of Aorta

Ascending aorta

Celiac trunk

Brachial a.

Ulnar a.

Radial artery

Posterior tibial artery

Anterior tibial artery

Fibular a.

Dorsal pedialis a.

FIGURE 17-2 Arteries of the Body

B. MAJOR VENOUS SUPPLY

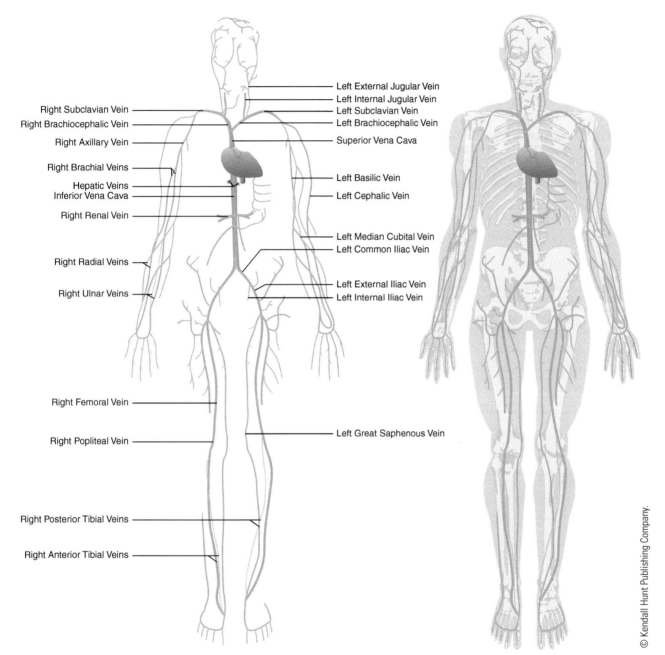

Right Subclavian Vein

Right Brachiocephalic Vein

Right Axillary Vein

Right Brachial Veins

Hepatic Veins
Inferior Vena Cava

Right Renal Vein

Right Radial Veins

Right Ulnar Veins

Right Femoral Vein

Right Popliteal Vein

Right Posterior Tibial Veins

Right Anterior Tibial Veins

Left External Jugular Vein
Left Internal Jugular Vein
Left Subclavian Vein
Left Brachiocephalic Vein

Superior Vena Cava

Left Basilic Vein

Left Cephalic Vein

Left Median Cubital Vein
Left Common Iliac Vein

Left External Iliac Vein
Left Internal Iliac Vein

Left Great Saphenous Vein

FIGURE 17-3 Major Veins—Anterior View

III. Lab Activity: Cardiovascular System: Blood Vessels

Identify the following cardiovascular blood vessel structures on the models

BLOOD VESSELS:

General Structures

- artery and vein (w/valves)
  - tunica externa (adventitia)
  - tunica media
  - elastic lamina
  - tunica interna (intima)

HEAD, NECK, AND ARMS AND ABDOMEN (SELECTED)

Arteries: Head, Neck

- aorta (ascending, arch, descending)
- aorta (thoracic)
- brachiocephalic (innominate)
- common carotid a.
- carotid sinus
- internal carotid a.
- external carotid a.
- superficial temporal a.
- subclavian a.
- vertebral a.
- internal thoracic (mammary) a.
- axillary
- circumflex humeral (anterior, posterior)
- brachial a.
- radial a.
- ulnar a.
- palmar arches: superficial/deep a.

Veins: Head, Neck/Arm

- superior vena cava
- brachiocephalic (innominate) veins: R&L
- internal jugular v.
- subclavian v.
- external jugular v.
- axillary v.
- cephalic v.
- basilic v.
- median cubital v.
- brachial v.
- radial v.
- ulnar v.

Selected Vessels of the Abdomen

Arteries

- abdominal aorta
- celiac trunk
- left gastric artery
- splenic artery
- common hepatic artery
- superior mesenteric artery
- inferior mesenteric artery
- renal artery
- gonadal artery
- common iliac artery
- internal iliac artery
- external iliac artery

Selected Vessels of the Abdomen

Veins

- inferior vena cava vein
- hepatic portal vein (and branches)
  - gastric veins
  - splenic vein
  - superior mesenteric vein
  - inferior mesenteric vein
- suprarenal vein
- renal vein
- gonadal vein
- common iliac vein
- internal iliac vein
- external iliac vein

VESSELS OF THE LEG ARTERIES

- internal iliac a.
- external iliac a.
- femoral a.
- popliteal a.
- anterior tibial a.
- posterior tibial a.

VESSELS OF THE LEG VEINS:

- internal iliac v.
- external iliac v.
- femoral v.

- great saphenous v.
- popliteal v.
- anterior tibial v.
- posterior tibial v.

IV. Vessels of Head-Neck

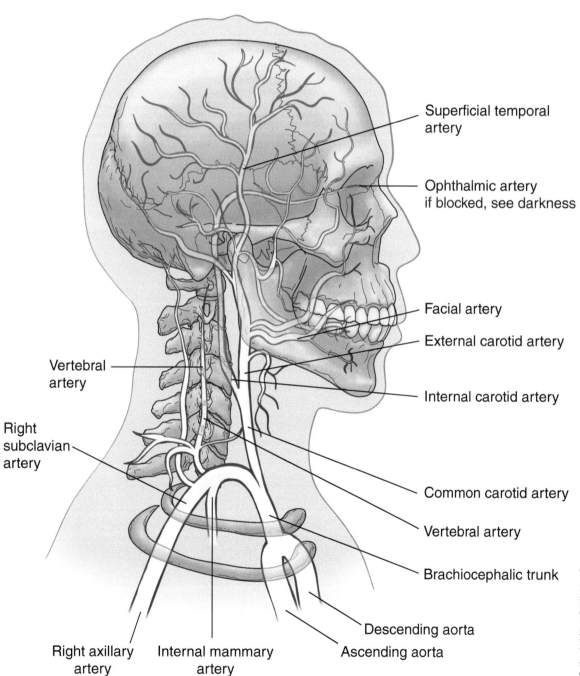

Superficial temporal artery

Ophthalmic artery
if blocked, see darkness

Facial artery

External carotid artery

Internal carotid artery

Common carotid artery

Vertebral artery

Brachiocephalic trunk

Descending aorta

Ascending aorta

Vertebral artery

Right subclavian artery

Right axillary artery

Internal mammary artery

FIGURE 17-4A Head/Neck Arteries: Right Side View

A. ARTERIAL DISTRIBUTION TO HEAD-NECK

TABLE 17-3 Systemic Arteries of the Neck and Head

ARTERY	AREA SUPPLIED
Brachiocephalic Trunk	Supplies vessels in the right arm and right side of the neck and head. Gives rise to the right common carotid and right subclavian arteries.
Common Carotid Arteries	Supplies the head and neck. Gives rise to the internal and external carotid arteries.
Internal Carotid Arteries	Supplies the brain and eye. Ends in terminal branches inside the cranium.
External Carotid Arteries	Supplies blood to the face and scalp. Gives rise to the superficial temporal and facial arteries.
Superficial Temporal Arteries	Supplies the superficial temporal scalp.
Vertebral Arteries	Supplies the brain and spinal cord. Joins to form the basilar artery at the base of the brain.

B. VENOUS DISTRIBUTION TO HEAD-NECK

TABLE 17-4 Systemic Veins of the Head and Neck

BLOOD VESSEL	DESCRIPTION
Brachiocephalic Veins	Drains the head and upper limbs. Short trunks unite to form the superior vena cava.
Internal Jugular Veins	Drains the brain, face, and neck. Travels inferiorly with the internal carotid and common carotid arteries. Joins the subclavian vein to form the brachiocephalic vein.
External Jugular Veins	Drains the superficial face, neck, and scalp. Ends at the subclavian vein.
Retromandibular Veins	Drains the superficial temporal scalp and face. Gives rise to the external jugular vein.
Superficial Temporal Veins	Drains the superficial temporal scalp. Gives rise to the retromandibular vein.
Vertebral Veins	Drains the brain and spinal cord. Ends at the subclavian vein.

C. LAB ACTVITY 1: LABEL THESE STRUCTURES

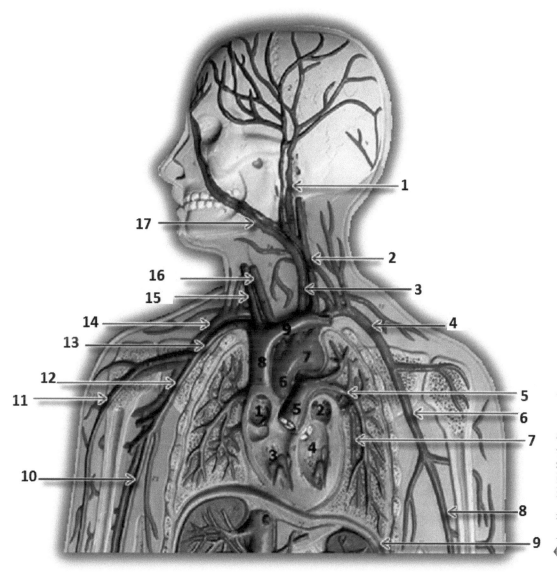

Item No. 1000276 [G30] - Circulatory System, © 3B Scientific GmbH, Germany, 2018, www.3bscientific.com. From *Anatomy and Physiology Laboratory Manual*, 5th Edition, by Carolyn Robertson et al. © Kendall Hunt Publishing Company.

FIGURE 17-4B

V. Cerebral Blood Flow (Circle of Willis)

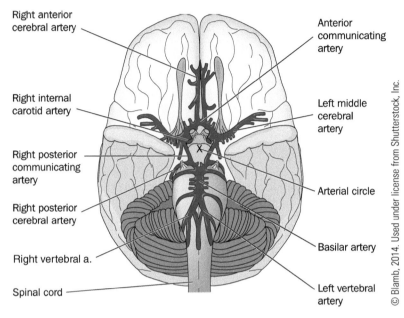

FIGURE 17-5 Circle of Willis

A. Formed primarily by two vessels: **vertebral and internal carotid arteries.**

B. **Vertebral arteries** (both right and left) take off from the subclavian arteries, ascend, and travel in the transverse foramen of the cervical vertebrae. Both unite at the level of the medulla oblongata forming the **basilar artery,** supplying the brain stem. They then join with the **internal carotid arteries, together** forming the network of arteries supplying the brain and brain stem called **Circle of Willis (cerebral arterial circle).**

C. **Internal carotid arteries** (right and left) take off of the common carotid artery, travel through the carotid canal, and then join with branches of the **vertebral arteries** to form the **Circle of Willis.**

D. **LAB ACTVITY 2:** LABEL THESE STRUCTURES

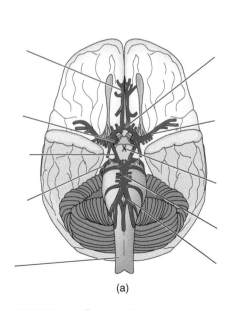

(a)

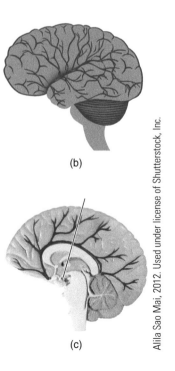

(b)

(c)

FIGURE 17-6 Cerebral Arteries

VI. Vessels of Upper Extremities

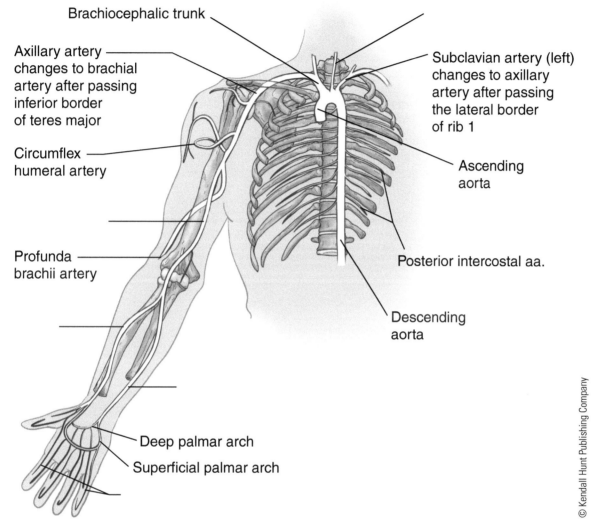

Brachiocephalic trunk

Axillary artery
changes to brachial
artery after passing
inferior border
of teres major

Subclavian artery (left)
changes to axillary
artery after passing
the lateral border
of rib 1

Circumflex
humeral artery

Ascending
aorta

Profunda
brachii artery

Posterior intercostal aa.

Descending
aorta

Deep palmar arch
Superficial palmar arch

FIGURE 17-7 Upper Limb Arteries

© Kendall Hunt Publishing Company

A. ARTERIAL DISTRIBUTION

TABLE 17-5 Systemic Arteries of the Upper Limbs

ARTERY	AREA SUPPLIED
Subclavian Arteries	Supplies blood to the upper limbs. Gives rise to the axillary and vertebral arteries.
Axillary Arteries	Continuation of the subclavian artery. Supplies blood to the shoulder. Gives rise to the brachial arteries.
Brachial Arteries	Continuation of the axillary artery. Supplies blood to the arm. Gives rise to the ulnar and radial arteries.
Radial Arteries	Supplies blood to the lateral side of the forearm. Gives rise to the superficial and deep palmar arches.
Ulnar Arteries	Supplies blood to the medial side of the forearm. Gives rise to the superficial and deep palmar arches.
Superficial Palmar Arches	Branch of the radial artery. Anastomoses with the ulnar artery. Supplies the digits.
Deep Palmar Arches	Branch of the ulnar artery. Anastomoses with the radial artery. Supplies the carpal bones.

B. VENOUS DISTRIBUTION

TABLE 17-6 Systemic Veins of the Upper Limbs

BLOOD VESSEL	DESCRIPTION
Subclavian Veins	Drains the upper extremities. Joins the internal jugular vein to form the brachiocephalic vein.
Axillary Veins	Drains the upper limbs. Begins at the junction of the basilic and brachial veins. Gives rise to the subclavian vein.
Brachial Veins	Drains the deep structures of the arms. Joins the basilica veins to form the axillary vein.
Radial Veins	Drains the deep structures of the lateral forearm. Joins the ulnar vein to form the brachial vein.
Ulnar Veins	Drains the deep structures of the medial forearm. Joins the radial vein to form the brachial vein.
Cephalic Veins	Drains the superficial structures of the lateral forearm. Has an anastomose with the median cubital vein and ends at the axillary vein.
Basilic Veins	Drains the superficial structures of the medial forearm. Joined by the median cubital vein before joining the brachial vein to form the axillary vein.
Median Cubital Veins	Drains the superficial median cubital fossa. Forms an anastomose between the cephalic, basilica, and several deep veins.
Superficial Palmar Venous Arch	Drains the digits and posterior region of the hand. Gives rise to the cephalic and basilic veins.
Deep Palmar Venous Arch	Drains the digits and anterior region of the hand. Gives rise to the radial and ulnar veins.

VII. Vessels of the Trunk

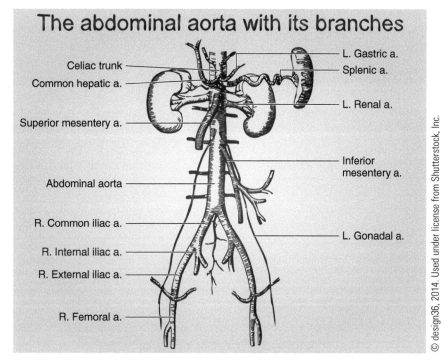

FIGURE 17-8 Abdominal Aorta Branches Labelled

A. ARTERIAL DISTRIBUTION

TABLE 17-7 Systemic Arteries of the Trunk

ARTERY	AREA SUPPLIED
Renal Arteries	Branches from the aorta immediately caudal to the superior mesenteric artery. Supplies the kidneys.
Celiac Trunk	Branches from the aorta inferior to the diaphragm. Gives rise to the gastric, splenic, and common hepatic arteries.
Gastric Artery	Branch of the celiac trunk. Supplies the stomach and esophagus.
Splenic Artery	Branch of the celiac trunk. Supplies the spleen, stomach, and pancreas.
Common Hepatic Artery	Branch of the celiac trunk. Supplies the stomach, liver, and gallbladder.
Superior Mesenteric Artery	Branches from the aorta inferior to the celiac trunk. Supplies the small intestine, appendix, and first half of the large intestine.
Inferior Mesenteric Artery	Branches from the aorta inferior to the superior mesenteric artery. Supplies the second half of the large intestine and rectum.

B. VENOUS DISTRIBUTION

TABLE 17-8 Systemic Veins of the Trunk

BLOOD VESSEL	DESCRIPTION
Renal Veins	Drains the kidneys. Empties directly into the inferior vena cava.
Hepatic Veins	Drains the hepatic sinusoids. Empties into the inferior vena cava.
Hepatic Sinusoids	Capillaries found in the liver. Unique as both arterial blood supplied by the hepatic artery and venous blood supplied by the hepatic portal vein are delivered.
Hepatic Portal Vein	Delivers blood to the liver from most of the abdominal organs. Formed by the junction of the superior mesenteric and splenic veins, and gastric veins.
Short Gastric Veins	Drains the fundus and the greater curvature of the stomach. Empties into the splenic vein.
Pyloric Vein	Drains the pylorus and lesser curvature of the stomach. Empties into the hepatic portal vein.
Cystic Vein	Drains the gallbladder. Empties into the hepatic portal vein.
Superior Mesenteric Vein	Drains the small intestine and first half of the large intestine. Joins the splenic vein to form the hepatic portal vein.
Splenic Vein	Drains the spleen, stomach, pancreas, and the second half of the large intestine. Joins the superior mesenteric vein to form the hepatic portal vein.
Pancreatic Veins	Drains the body and tail of the pancreas. Empties into the splenic vein.
Inferior Mesenteric Vein	Drains the second half of the large intestine. Empties into the splenic vein.

C. HEPATIC PORTAL SYSTEM

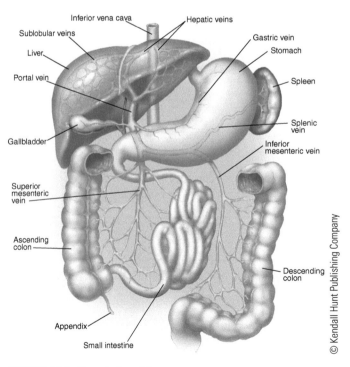

FIGURE 17-9 Hepatic Portal System

D. LAB ACTVITY 4: LABEL THESE STRUCTURES

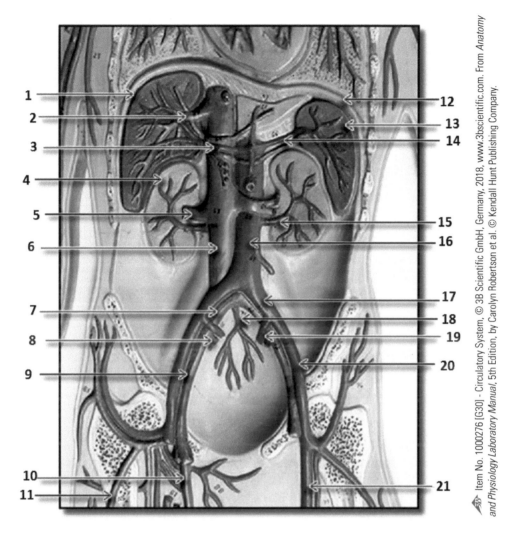

Item No. 1000276 [G30] - Circulatory System, © 3B Scientific GmbH, Germany, 2018, www.3bscientific.com. From *Anatomy and Physiology Laboratory Manual*, 5th Edition, by Carolyn Robertson et al. © Kendall Hunt Publishing Company.

FIGURE 17-10 Abdominal Pelvic Vessels

VIII. Vessels of the Lower Extremities

A. ARTERIAL DISTRIBUTION

TABLE 17-9 Systemic Arteries of the Lower Limbs

ARTERY	AREA SUPPLIED
Common Iliac Arteries	Rises from the bifurcation of the distal portion of the aorta. Gives rise to the internal and external iliac arteries.
External Iliac Arteries	Branch of the common iliac artery. Supplies blood to the lower limb. Gives rise to the femoral artery.
Internal Iliac Arteries	Branch of the common iliac artery. Supplies blood to the viscera of the pelvic and gluteal regions.
Femoral Arteries	Continuation of the external iliac artery. Supplies blood to the thigh. Gives rise to the popliteal arteries.
Popliteal Arteries	Continuation of the femoral artery. Supplies blood to the posterior knee. Gives rise to the anterior and posterior tibial arteries.
Anterior Tibial Arteries	Branch of the popliteal artery. Supplies the anterior lower leg. Gives rise to the dorsalis pedis artery.
Posterior Tibial Arteries	Branch of the popliteal artery. Supplies the posterior lower leg.
Dorsalis Pedis Arteries	Continuation of the anterior tibial artery. Supplies the ankle foot.

B. VENOUS DISTRIBUTION

TABLE 17-10 Systemic Veins of the Lower Limbs

BLOOD VESSEL	DESCRIPTION
Common Iliac Vein	Drains the pelvis and lower limbs. Joins together at the distal bifurcation of the inferior vena cava.
Internal Iliac Veins	Drains the pelvis. Joins the external iliac vein to form the common iliac vein.
External Iliac Veins	Drains the lower limb. Joins the internal iliac vein to form the common iliac vein.
Femoral Veins	Drains the lower limb. Joins the great saphenous vein to form the external iliac vein.
Great Saphenous Vein	Drains the superficial medial side of the foot, leg, knee, and thigh. Joins the femoral vein to form the external iliac vein. Longest vein in the body.
Popliteal Veins	Drains the knee and lower leg. Formed by the anterior and posterior tibial veins.
Anterior Tibial Veins	Drains the anterior lower leg. Joins the posterior tibial vein to form the popliteal vein.
Posterior Tibial Veins	Drains the posterior lower leg. Joins the anterior tibial vein to form the popliteal vein.
Dorsal Venous Arch	Drains the ankle and foot. Continues to form the great saphenous vein.
Deep Plantar Arch	Drains the plantar surface of the foot. Continues to form the posterior tibial vein.

C. LAB ACTIVITY 5: LABEL THESE STRUCTURES

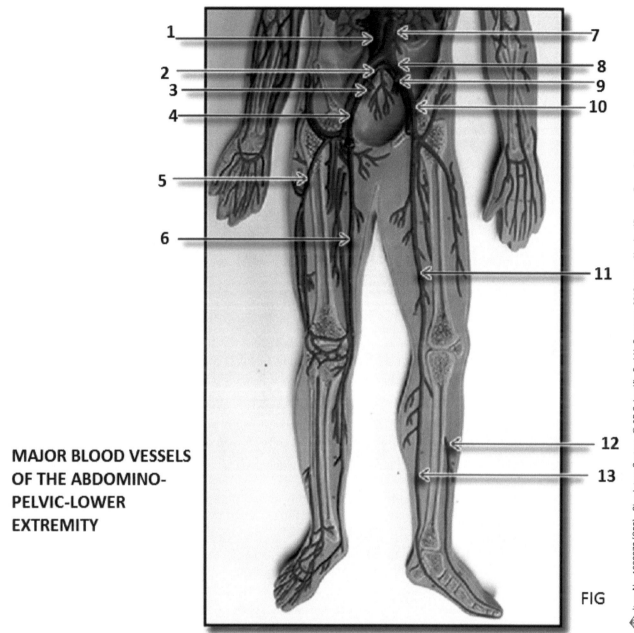

MAJOR BLOOD VESSELS
OF THE ABDOMINO-
PELVIC-LOWER
EXTREMITY

Item No. 1000276 [G30] - Circulatory System, © 3B Scientific GmbH, Germany, 2018, www.3bscientific.com. From *Anatomy and Physiology Laboratory Manual*, 5th Edition, by Carolyn Robertson et al. © Kendall Hunt Publishing Company.

FIGURE 17-11 Major Blood Vessels, Lower Body

IX. Fetal Circulation

A. During intrauterine life, the fetal respiratory and digestive systems are not totally functional yet. Therefore, nutrient supply and waste removal are dependent on the placental vessels that carry these to and from the fetus.

B.

TABLE 17-11 Fetal Circulation

FETAL STRUCTURE	FEATURES/INTRAUTERINE FUNCTIONS	REMNANT STRUCTURE (AFTER BIRTH)
PLACENTA	Connects the maternal uterine wall to the fetus. A semipermeable membrane barrier allows for gaseous and nutrient supply to the developing fetus plus waste material from the baby to the placenta.	**DISCARDED**
UMBILICAL CORD	From the placenta to the baby. Has 3 vessels: 2 arteries and 1 vein.	**DISCARDED WITH PLACENTA**
UMBILICAL ARTERIES (2)	The 2 arteries originate from the internal iliac arteries and carry deoxygenated blood/waste from fetus to the placenta.	**2 LATERAL UMBILICAL LIGAMENTS**
UMBILICAL VEIN (1)	This vein carries oxygenated blood from the placental to the fetal inferior vena cava (IVC) and then subsequently to the right atrium (RA)	**ROUND LIGAMENT (Ligamentum Teres) OF THE LIVER**
DUCTUS VENOSUS (1 OF 3 SHUNTS)	This structure bypasses (flow through) the liver and directly into the IVC.	**LIGAMENTUM VENOSUS**
FORAMEN OVALE (2 OF 3 SHUNTS)	Number 1 of 2 structures that shunts (bypasses) blood from the nonfunctioning lungs in the fetus. Located in the atrial septum. Carries blood from the RA to the left atrium (LA), bypassing most of the flow to the right ventricle that would have otherwise ended up in the lungs.	**FOSSA OVALE OF ATRIA SEPTUM**
DUCTUS ARTERIOSUS (3 OF 3 SHUNTS)	Number 2 of 2 structures that shunts (bypasses) blood from the nonfunctioning lungs in the fetus. Located between the pulmonary artery and the aorta. Carries blood from the pulmonary artery (trunk) to the arch of the aorta, bypassing the lungs totally.	**LIGAMENTUM ARTERIOSUS**

C.

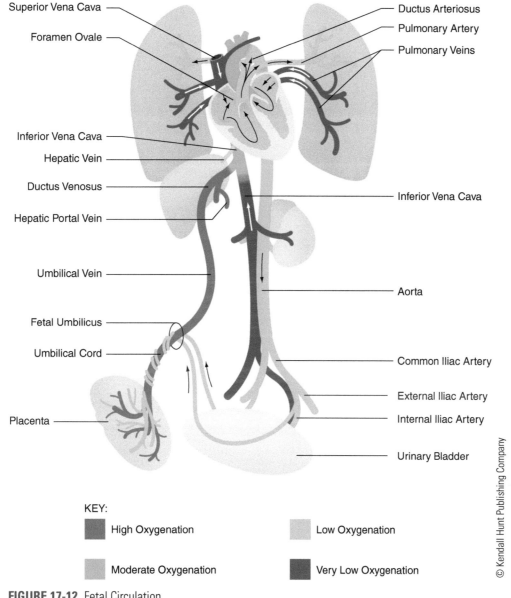

FIGURE 17-12 Fetal Circulation

X. Pulse Point Determination

A.

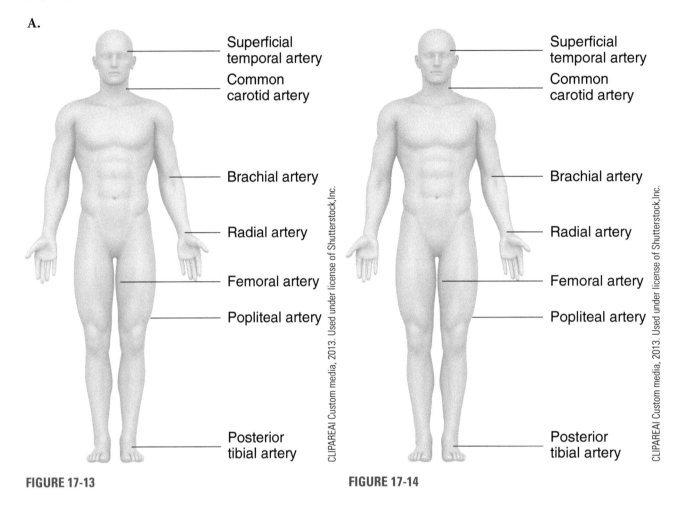

Superficial temporal artery

Common carotid artery

Brachial artery

Radial artery

Femoral artery

Popliteal artery

Posterior tibial artery

CLIPAREAI Custom media, 2013. Used under license of Shutterstock,Inc.

Superficial temporal artery

Common carotid artery

Brachial artery

Radial artery

Femoral artery

Popliteal artery

Posterior tibial artery

CLIPAREAI Custom media, 2013. Used under license of Shutterstock,Inc.

FIGURE 17-13

FIGURE 17-14

XI. Clinical Applications on Blood Vessels

A.

TABLE 17-12 Clinical Applications on Blood Vessels

DISEASE/CONDITION	DEFINITION/SYMPTOMS	DIAGNOSIS/TREATMENT
ANEURYSM	Dilated weakened blood vessel due to hypertension or congenital. No symptoms until ruptured.	Sonogram, angiogram. Surgical repair.
ATHEROSCLEROSIS	Atheroma (plaque) formed within arteries. Hypertension and ischemia, coronary disease, stroke, death.	Drug therapy +/- surgery.
ARTERIOSCLEROSIS	Hardening of the arteries and scarring ("sclerosis"), loss of wall flexibility. Hypertension, coronary disease, stroke, death.	Drug therapy +/- surgery.
HYPERTENSION	Unknown or second to atherosclerosis. Silent killer. Elevated BP.	BP monitor and control: exercise, drug treatment.
THROMBOPHLEBITIS	Painful, inflamed, swollen extremity due to thrombus (clot) formation.	Physical exam, Doppler sonogram. Anticoagulants, antibiotics +/- surgery.
VARICOSE VEINS	Due to excess weight, prolonged standing. Swollen of veins. Cosmetic spider veins or hemorrhoids.	Compression stockings, surgery or sclerotherapy.

XII. Pre-Lab Activity: Blood Vessels

A. Fill-in-the-blank

1. List the three layers of a blood vessel from superficial to deep:

   i. _____

   ii. _____

   iii. _____

2. _____ are the smallest arteries in diameter delivering blood to the capillaries.

3. List the three types of capillaries from most permeable to least permeable:

   i. _____

   ii. _____

   iii. _____

4. _____ represents the force exerted by the left ventricle.

5. _____ is the instrument placed around the arm to get a blood pressure reading.

6. List the four major pulse points on the human body:

   i. _____

   ii. _____

   iii. _____

   iv. _____

7. _____ is the rhythmic expansion and recoil of the arteries.

8. The _____ supplies oxygenated blood to the kidneys.

9. The _____ drains deoxygenated blood from the stomach.

XIII. Post-Lab Activity: Heart

A. LABEL THESE DIAGRAMS:

I)

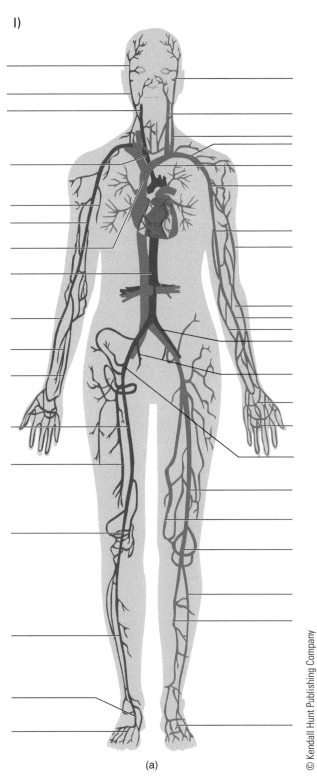

(a)

FIGURE 17-15 Blood Vessels

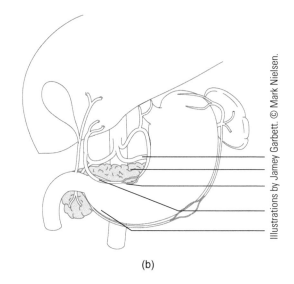

(b)

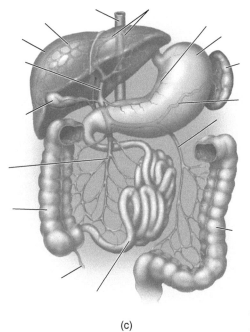

(c)

Illustrations by Jamey Garbett. © Mark Nielsen.

© Kendall Hunt Publishing Company

© Kendall Hunt Publishing Company

II)

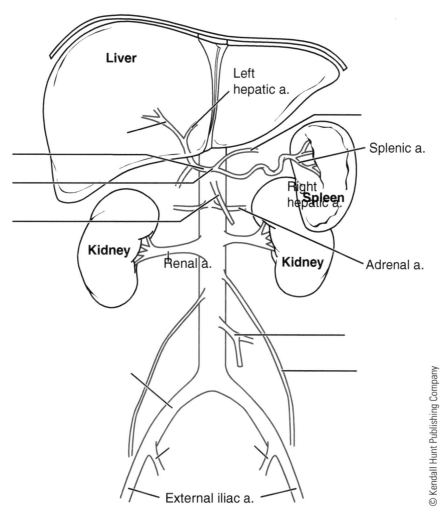

Liver

Left
hepatic a.

Splenic a.

Right
hepatic a.

Spleen

Kidney

Renal a.

Kidney

Adrenal a.

External iliac a.

FIGURE 17-16 Abdominal Arteries

B. Answer the following:

1. This vein is considered the longest vein in the human body:
   A. femoral vein
   B. small saphenous vein
   C. great saphenous vein
   D. inferior vena cava

2. All absorbed nutrients (postabsorption) from the digestive tract enter this vessel:
   A. hepatic vein
   B. splenic vein
   C. hepatic portal vein
   D. inferior vena cava

3. All venous drainage from the brain toward the heart drains into this vessel:
   A. external jugular
   B. internal jugular
   C. subclavian vein
   D. axillary vein

4. Which of the following are branches off of the aortic arch?
    A. right and left common carotid arteries
    B. left subclavian artery and left common carotid artery
    C. right brachial and left axillary arteries
    D. right and left subclavian arteries

5. Compare and contrast the anatomy of the artery and vein structure.

6. List the two structures that have valves in the human body.

7. Distinguish between atherosclerosis and arteriosclerosis.

Lymphatic System

Upon completion of this exercise, you should be able to:

A. Identify the organs of the lymphatic system including functions.
B. Identify the mucosae-associated lymphatic tissues (MALT) in the lymphatic system with their anatomical features, location in the body, and function.
C. Describe the basic structure and cellular composition of lymphatic tissue and correlate it to the overall functions of the lymphatic system.
D. Describe the lymphatic drainage system.
E. Describe the roles of various types of leukocytes in innate and adaptive body defenses.
F. List the clinical applications.

NEEDED MATERIALS

1. Lymphatic wall plaque (Model).
2. Human torso with deep blood vessels of the thorax and upper abdomen.

Introduction

I. OVERVIEW

A. The **lymphatic system** consists of lymph (fluid), lymphatic vessels, lymphoid tissue, and lymphoid organs.
B. **Lymph** is the excess fluid (plasma minus proteins) leaked from around capillaries surrounding organs—all that are not picked up by the venous drainage.
C. **FUNCTIONS:** The lymphatic system has a dual function in:
   A. **Immunity:** Responsible for either the manufacture or development and housing of cells of immunity (lymphocytes).
   B. **Fluid balance:** Collecting leaked fluid (lymph) as much as 2 to 3 L/day from around tissues/organs and returning them to the circulatory system.
D. **Lymphatic capillaries** (similar to and surround blood capillaries around organs) collect excess/linked fluid (lymph) and become lymphatic vessels.
E. **Lymphatic vessels** collect lymph fluid from capillaries and drain into larger collecting vessels/ducts or into regional lymph nodes. They have valves (to prevent back flow) similar to veins.
F. **Lymphatic nodes** are found in groups in different regions—cervical group, axillary group, and inguinal group of nodes. They are house-specific and nonspecific cells of immunity and the only structure that would filter antigens.
G. **Cisterna chyli** is located in the upper abdomen and receives lymph drainage from the lower extremities and lower abdomen. The thoracic duct takes off from this.
H. **Thoracic duct** originates in the upper abdomen from the **cisterna chili,** and ascends to the left side in the thorax while eventually draining into the **left subclavian vein.**
   It is responsible for the lymphatic drainage of lower extremities, lower trunk/abdomen, left upper trunk, left upper extremity, and left head-neck areas because smaller lymphatic vessels from these area drain into it before entering the left subclavian vein.
I. **Right lymphatic duct** originates from the collection of several smaller lymphatic vessels draining the right arm, right upper trunk, and right head-neck. It eventually drains into the **right subclavian vein.**
   It is responsible for the lymphatic drainage of right arm, right upper trunk, and right head-neck areas.

J. **Major lymphoid organs** are divided into two groups:
   1. **Primary lymphoid organs** are responsible for the manufacture or maturation of lymphocytes (B and T): **bone marrow and thymus.**
   2. **Secondary lymphoid organs/tissues** are the house (and clone site) for lymphocytes, memory cells, and other nonspecific cells of immunity. They also include spleen, lymph nodes, tonsils, and lymphoid tissues such as MALT.
K. **Mucosae-associated lymphatic tissues** are part of the lymphatic system. They are found in the mucosal areas of **respiratory tract, gastrointestinal tract (as Peyer patches), appendix, and urinary tract.** Helps trap antigens before they can enter the blood.

TABLE 18-1 Primary vs Secondary Lymphoid Organs

PRIMARY LYMPHOID ORGANS	SECONDARY LYMPHOID ORGANS
Ex: Bone Marrow, Thymus	Ex: Spleen, Nodes, Malt (Peyer's Patches, Appendix), Tonsils
■ Lymphoid stem cells proliferate & mature	■ Lymphoid cells become functional
■ Contain B or T lymphocytes	■ Contain B & T Lymphocytes
■ Antigens cannot enter	■ Antigens enter
■ Atrophy with age □ (thymus only, not bone marrow)	■ Enlarge with age

TABLE 18-2 Different Types of Immune Cells

CELL	DESCRIPTION
T-Lymphocytes	(T cells) Make up approximately 80% of circulating lymphocytes. Produced in the thymus; responsible for attacking and destroying foreign cells (direct cellular immunity).
Helper T Cells	Special type of T cell that stimulates the functions of both T cells and B cells.
B-Lymphocytes	(B cells) Make up approximately 10–15% of circulating lymphocytes. Produced in the bone marrow; differentiate into plasma cells after exposure to specific antigens.
Plasma Cells	Produce antibodies which target specific antigens (antibody-mediated immunity).
Natural Killer Cells	Make up 5–10% of circulating lymphocytes. NK cells are responsible for immunological surveillance and attacking foreign cells, virus-infected cells, and cancer cells.
Macrophages	Phagocytizes bacteria and helps activate T cells.
Reticular Cells	Binds to antigens and presents them to other immune cells.
Dendritic Cells	Forms the stroma (structural network that supports other immune cells) in most lymph organs.

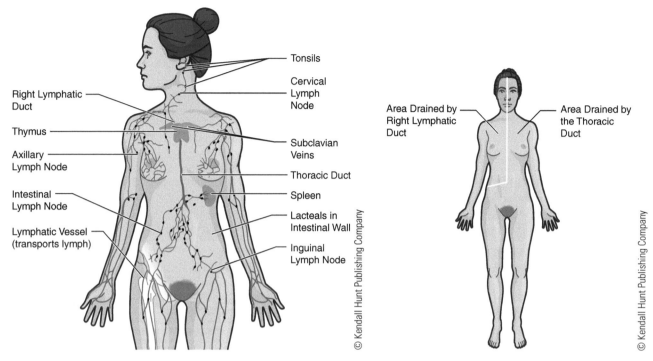

Tonsils

Cervical Lymph Node

Right Lymphatic Duct

Thymus

Axillary Lymph Node

Subclavian Veins

Thoracic Duct

Spleen

Intestinal Lymph Node

Lacteals in Intestinal Wall

Lymphatic Vessel (transports lymph)

Inguinal Lymph Node

© Kendall Hunt Publishing Company

FIGURE 18-1A Lympathic system-left superior body

Area Drained by Right Lymphatic Duct

Area Drained by the Thoracic Duct

© Kendall Hunt Publishing Company

FIGURE 18-1B Lympathic system-right superior body

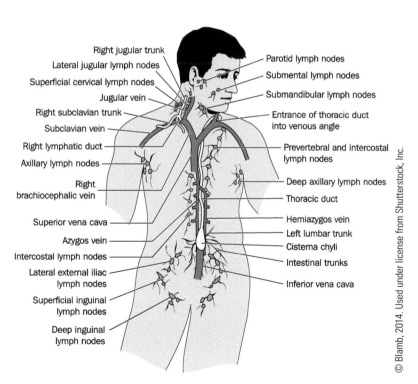

Right jugular trunk

Lateral jugular lymph nodes

Superficial cervical lymph nodes

Jugular vein

Right subclavian trunk

Subclavian vein

Right lymphatic duct

Axillary lymph nodes

Right brachiocephalic vein

Superior vena cava

Azygos vein

Intercostal lymph nodes

Lateral external iliac lymph nodes

Superficial inguinal lymph nodes

Deep inguinal lymph nodes

Parotid lymph nodes

Submental lymph nodes

Submandibular lymph nodes

Entrance of thoracic duct into venous angle

Prevertebral and intercostal lymph nodes

Deep axillary lymph nodes

Thoracic duct

Hemiazygos vein

Left lumbar trunk

Cisterna chyli

Intestinal trunks

Inferior vena cava

© Blamb, 2014. Used under license from Shutterstock, Inc.

FIGURE 18-2 Diagram of Lymphatic & Drainage

II. Clinical Applications

TABLE 18-3 Clinical Applications

Human Immunodeficiency Virus (HIV): Disease that targets the helper T cells. With progression to acquired immune deficiency syndrome (AIDS), the lack of helper T cells suppresses the immune system and compromises an individual's ability to fight off secondary infections.
Lymphadenopathy: Enlargement or swelling of the lymph nodes caused by a number of diseases.
Edema: (*lymphedema*) Blockage of normal lymph drainage leading to swelling associated with the accumulation of fluid. Can be temporarily caused by tight fitting clothing or sleeping incorrectly. It can also be *filariasis*, a disease caused by a parasitic roundworm belonging to the family *filariae*. Extreme tissue swelling of the limbs and genitalia caused by these worms is called *elephantiasis*.
Autoimmune disease: Malfunction in the immune system where an *autoimmune response* is triggered and the immune system begins to create antibodies against the body's own tissue.
Buboes: Swelling of the lymph nodes in response to infections such as bubonic plague, gonorrhea, tuberculosis, or syphilis.
Tonsillitis: Inflammation of the tonsils caused by either viral or bacterial infection. If the condition becomes chronic, a *tonsillectomy* can be performed to remove the tonsils completely or partially.

III. Lab Activity 18-1: Identify the Structures on the Lymphatic System

See Photos Atlas

TABLE 18-4 Lymphatic System

■ lymph node
■ regional lymph nodes: cervical, axillary, inguinal
■ cisterna chyli
■ thoracic duct
■ right lymphatic duct
■ thymus
■ spleen
■ lymphatic vessels (w/ valves)
■ azygos vein
■ hemiazygos vein
■ subclavian veins (R and L)

III. Lab Activity 18-2A: Activity Labeling

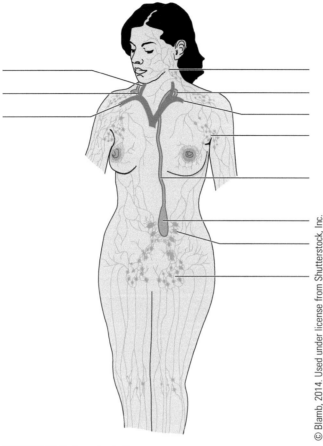

FIGURE 18-3 Lymphatic System

IV. Lab Activity Blood Vessels and Lymphatic System

Practice Quiz

1. Choose the correct pathway.
   A. Blood capillary → lymphatic capillary → efferent vessel → lymph node → afferent vessel → vein
   B. Blood capillary → lymphatic capillary → lymph node → afferent vessel → efferent vessel → vein
   C. Blood capillary → lymphatic capillary → afferent vessel → lymph node → efferent vessel → artery
   D. Blood capillary → lymphatic capillary → afferent vessel → lymph node → efferent vessel → vein
   E. Blood capillary → lymphatic capillary → lymph node → efferent vessel → afferent vessel → artery

2. The afferent lymphatic vessel does all of the following EXCEPT:
   A. Allows lymph to flow through
   B. Has valves
   C. Has a structure that allows lymph to flow in 2 directions
   D. Sends lymph to an artery

3. Using the diagram at the bottom of this page, choose the correct statement.
   A. E drains all of the neck, axilla, and groin
   B. AE drains into the left subclavian vein
   C. C drains into the left subclavian and left internal jugular vein
   D. E drains the entire head and neck
   E. The right upper limb is drained by C

4. The duct that drains AD

5. The duct that drains AE

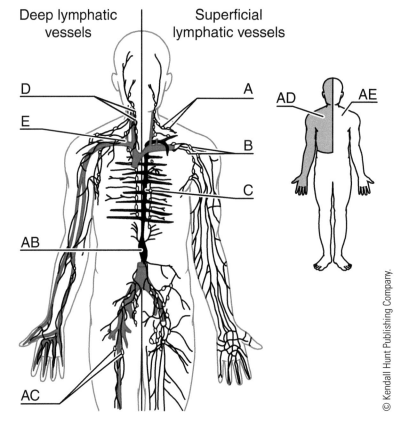

Deep lymphatic vessels   Superficial lymphatic vessels

D
E
A
AD
AE
B
C
AB
AC

© Kendall Hunt Publishing Company.

FIGURE 18-4

V. Complete the following

1. The largest lymphatic organ is the
   A. spleen
   B. tonsils
   C. thymus
   D. lymph nodes

2. Which of the following is considered a primary lymphatic organ?
   A. spleen
   B. thymus gland
   C. Peyer patches
   D. lymph nodes

3. Antibody production is a function of these cells:

   A. mast cells

   B. monocytes

   C. plasma cells

   D. neutrophils

4. Cellular immunity is attributed to this group of cells:

   A. Plasma cells

   B. T lymphocytes

   C. B lymphocytes

   D. macrophages

5. After production and release from the bone marrow, T lymphocytes must mature in which of the listed lymphoid organs mentioned below?

   A. thymus

   B. spleen

   C. lymph nodes

   D. bones

6. Lymphatic drainage of the left side of the head, neck, trunk, and lower extremities is attributed to

   A. right lymphatic duct

   B. left lymphatic duct

   C. thoracic duct

   D. cisternal chyli

7. Peyer patches are located in the

   A. the spleen

   B. small intestine mucosa wall

   C. thymus

   D. lymph nodes

8. The thoracic lymphatic duct returns lymph into the cardiovascular system at the vessel:

   A. internal jugular vein

   B. external jugular vein

   C. right subclavian vein

   D. left subclavian vein

Respiratory System

LEARNING OUTCOMES

Upon completion of this exercise, you should be able to:

A. Describe the sequence of respiratory structures that air must pass through during inspiration.
B. Describe the structure and function(s) of the following: nasal cavities, paranasal sinuses, pharynx, larynx, trachea, bronchi, lungs, pleural membranes, pulmonary blood vessels and nerves, thoracic and pleural cavities, and diaphragm.
C. Describe the structure and role of the larynx of respiratory system in producing speech.
D. Name the three cell types (and function) found in alveoli, and the respiratory membrane.
E. Identify the muscles of respiration.
E. Compare and contrast the conducting and respiratory zones of the respiratory tract.
F. List the clinical applications.

NEEDED MATERIALS

1. Human torso: thorax.
2. Lung model.
3. Larynx model.
4. Sagittal (median) head-neck model.
5. Alveolar model.

Introduction

OVERVIEW

A. The respiratory system includes the upper respiratory structures (nasal cavity to the level of the larynx) and the lower respiratory structures to the level of the functional alveoli.

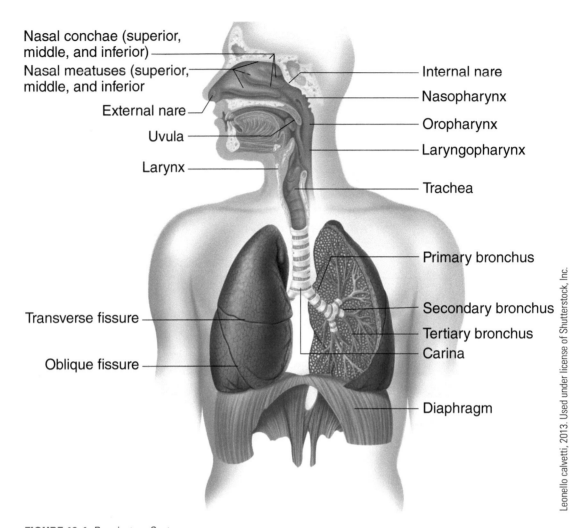

Nasal conchae (superior, middle, and inferior)
Nasal meatuses (superior, middle, and inferior
External nare
Uvula
Larynx
Internal nare
Nasopharynx
Oropharynx
Laryngopharynx
Trachea
Primary bronchus
Transverse fissure
Secondary bronchus
Tertiary bronchus
Carina
Oblique fissure
Diaphragm

Leonello calvetti, 2013. Used under license of Shutterstock, Inc.

FIGURE 19-1 Respiratory System

B. In addition to gaseous exchange, this system performs multiple functions, including but not limited to the following:

1. pH regulation: by controlling the level of carbon dioxide in the blood.

2. Voice production.

3. Production of angiotensin-converting enzyme (ACE) that converts angiotensinogen to angiotensin I, which is eventually converted by the kidneys to angiotensin II (AG II). AG II is the most powerful vasoconstrictor in the human body.

4. Olfactory (smell) function.

I. Upper Respiratory Track

TABLE 19-1 Upper Respiratory Structures

STRUCTURE	FEATURES/FUNCTION(S)
NASAL CAVITY	Filters and warms air.
PARANASAL SINUSES	Air-filled chambers of the skull; function primarily in the resonance of speech and include the following: **frontal, ethmoid, sphenoid, and maxillary.**
TONSILS	Aggregate of lymphoid tissues for airway immunity. Includes pharyngeal, palatine, and lingual tonsils. Additional mucosae-associated lymphatic tissues (MALT) are also found deeper in the lower respiratory system.
PHARYNX	Consists of 3 segments: nasopharynx, oropharynx, and laryngopharynx.
■ NASOPHARYNX	Part of the pharynx posterior to the nasal cavity. For air passage only. Located here is the pharyngotympanic (Eustachian) tube opening. Pharyngeal tonsils are located here.
■ OROPHARYNX	Part of the pharynx posterior to the oral cavity. For both air and food passage. Palatine tonsils are located here.
■ LARYNGOPHARYNX	Part of the pharynx posterior to the larynx. Allow for both air and food passage. Becomes the esophagus posterior to the larynx.

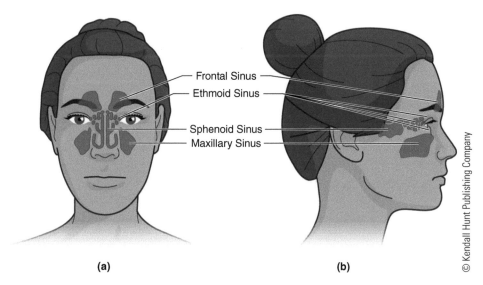

(a)   **(b)**

© Kendall Hunt Publishing Company

FIGURE 19-2 Paranasal Sinuses

II. Larynx

TABLE 19-2 Lower Respiratory Tract: The Larynx

STRUCTURE	FEATURES/FUNCTION(S)
LARYNX	Also known as "voice box," composed of 9 cartilages and 2 vocal ligaments. Connects the laryngopharynx above and the trachea below.
	Cartilages: 3 unpaired (epiglottis, thyroid, and cricoid) plus 3-paired small ones (arytenoids, cuneiform, and corniculate) located and embedded posteriorly.
HYOID BONE	Located in the neck superiorly to the thyroid cartilage. The thyro-hyoid membrane joins these 2 structures. Only bone in the body that do not attach to other bones. Serves as attachment for suprahyoid and infrahyoid muscles that move the larynx.
THYROID CARTILAGE	The largest cartilage forms the anterior-lateral wall of the larynx. Forms the laryngeal prominence anteriorly.
CRICOID CARTILAGE	Forms the inferior boundary of the larynx, attached to the thyroid superiorly via the crico-thyroid membrane.
EPIGLOTTIS	Made of elastic cartilage. Covers the glottis, prevents food into airways. As a result, food travels in the structure lying just posteriorly (esophagus) to the laryngopharynx.
OTHER CARTILAGES	3-paired small cartilages (arytenoid, cuneiform, and corniculate) forming the posterior pharynx.
GLOTTIS	The opening between the 2 true vocal ligaments. Leads from the laryngopharynx to the trachea lumen.
VOCAL CORD (FOLD)	Also known as true vocal cord/ligament. Made up of 2 ligaments attached to thyroid and the corniculate cartilages. Speech: air rushing from lungs through the glottis opening between the 2 vocal ligaments forms speech.
VESTIBULAR FOLD	Also called the false vocal fold. A mucosa fold above the true vocal cord. Not used for speech.
THYRO-HYOID MEMBRANE/LIGAMENT	Attaches the thyroid cartilage to the hyoid bone above.
CRICO-THYROID MEMBRANE/LIGAMENT	Attaches both the thyroid and cricoid cartilages. Often used in emergency to create a cricoidotomy (tube-like structure) for assistance in oxygen supply when the oral–tracheal intubation is impossible as in multiple facial/oral/basal fractures or injuries.
TRACHEAL RINGS	Located below the larynx. C-shaped, located posteriorly are the **trachealis muscles**. These smooth muscles cover the ends of the c-cartilages and when stimulated they contract to decrease tracheal lumen diameter as in forceful expulsion as in shouting/coughing.

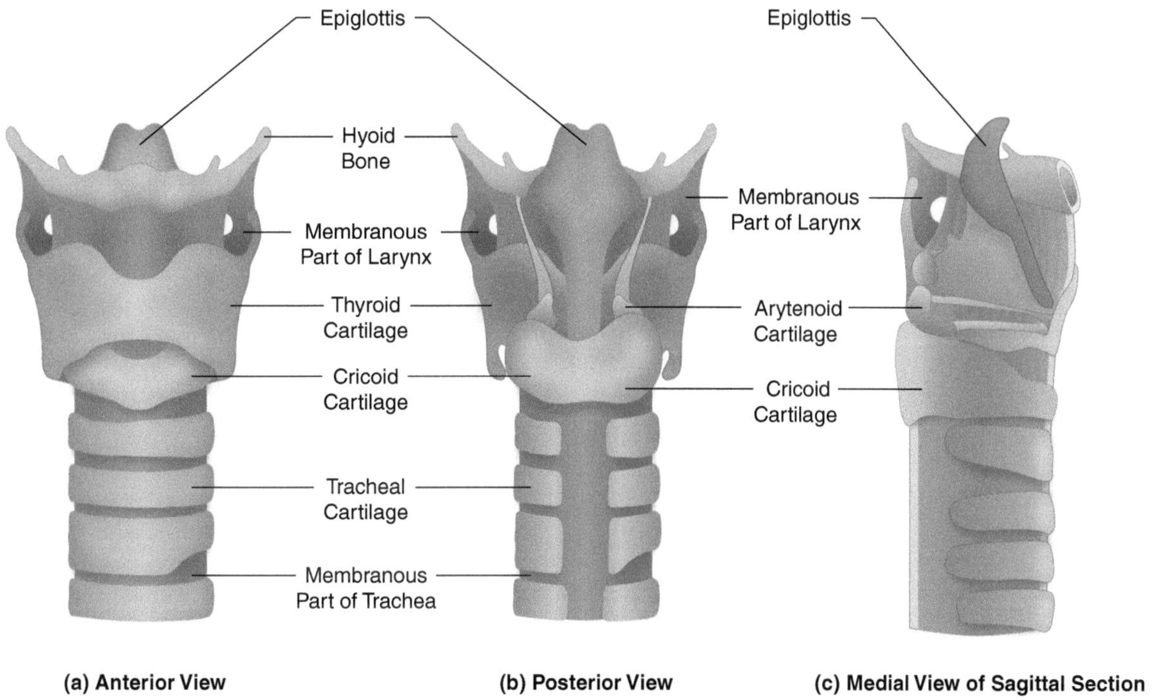

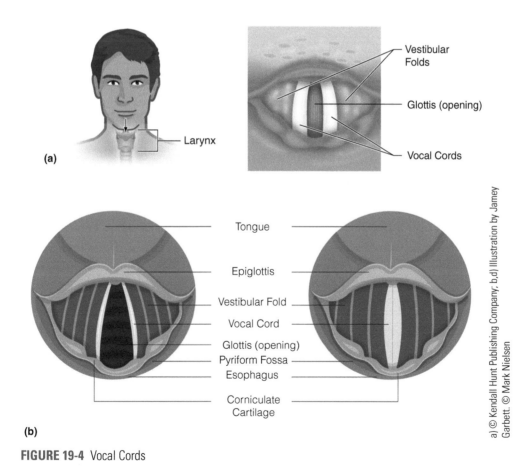

Epiglottis

Hyoid
Bone

Membranous
Part of Larynx

Thyroid
Cartilage

Cricoid
Cartilage

Tracheal
Cartilage

Membranous
Part of Trachea

(a) Anterior View

Epiglottis

Membranous
Part of Larynx

Arytenoid
Cartilage

Cricoid
Cartilage

(b) Posterior View

Epiglottis

(c) Medial View of Sagittal Section

© Kendall Hunt Publishing Company

FIGURE 19-3 Larynx

Larynx

(a)

Vestibular
Folds

Glottis (opening)

Vocal Cords

Tongue

Epiglottis

Vestibular Fold

Vocal Cord

Glottis (opening)

Pyriform Fossa

Esophagus

Corniculate
Cartilage

(b)

a) © Kendall Hunt Publishing Company; b,d) Illustration by Jamey
Garbett. © Mark Nielsen

FIGURE 19-4 Vocal Cords

III. Lower Respiratory Tract

TABLE 19-3 Lower Respiratory Structures

STRUCTURE	FEATURES/FUNCTION(S)
LARYNX	Also known as "voice box," composed of 9 cartilages in number and 2 vocal ligaments. Connects the laryngopharynx above and the trachea below. Cartilages: 3 unpaired (epiglottis, thyroid, and cricoid) plus 3-paired small ones (arytenoids, cuneiform, and corniculate) located and embedded posteriorly.
TRACHEA	Located below the larynx. C-shaped, located posteriorly are the **trachealis muscles**.
PLEURAL MEMBRANES	The pleurae (2) are the serous membranes covering the lung. Made up of fibrous outer **parietal pleural** that is also continuous with parietal pericardium, lines the thoracic walls. And a thinner **visceral pleura** that clings to the substance of the lung, dips into the fissure.
PLEURAL SPACE	
BRONCHI	Rigid air conducting tubes. **Primary/Main (2):** Right and left are outside the lungs and are formed from the bifurcation of the trachea. Left primary is longer but narrower. Right primary is shorter but wider. These further divide into secondary bronchi, etc. **Secondary (lobar), tertiary (segmental), and subsequent terminal (lobular) bronchioles** are referred to collectively as intrapulmonary bronchi (within the lung).
BRONCHIOLES	Terminal bronchioles have non-respiratory function (which are conducting tubes), whereas respiratory bronchioles (which give rise to alveoli ducts) have respiratory function.
CARINA	Last cartilage at the bifurcation of the trachea as it divides forming the 2 primary bronchi.
ALVEOLUS	The basic (smallest) functional unit of the lung. Clusters of alveoli are called alveoli sac and are surrounded by blood capillaries and elastin fibers. Exchange of gases takes place between the alveoli and capillaries.
ALVEOLI DUCT	A small tube between the respiratory bronchioles and the alveoli.
ALVEOLI SAC	A bunch collection of alveoli.
ALVEOLAR MACROPHAGES	1 of the 3 cell types that make up the alveolus. Also "dust cell," responsible for immunity.
LUNG FISSURES AND LOBES	**LEFT:** Divided into 2 lobes, superior and inferior, by oblique fissure. **RIGHT:** Divided into 3 lobes by 2 fissures: Oblique fissure (similar to left) but separates right middle and inferior lobes. Horizontal fissure separates superior right middle lobe.
RESPIRATORY MEMBRANE	Exchange of gases takes place here. A very thin complex composed of 3 structures: 1. Alveolar simple squamous epithelium on one side. 2. Capillary endothelium (simple squamous) on the other side plus. 3. Their basement membranes fused together in the middle.
TYPE I CELLS	2 of the 3 cell types that make up the alveolus. The wall of the each alveolus is made up of simple squamous epithelium (Type I). Allow for gaseous exchange with the surrounding capillaries.
TYPE II CELLS	3 of the 3 cell types that make up the alveolus and are much fewer than the Type I cells. Type II cells produce surfactants, which are responsible for preventing the alveoli from collapsing on self.

Bronchial Tree Up-Close

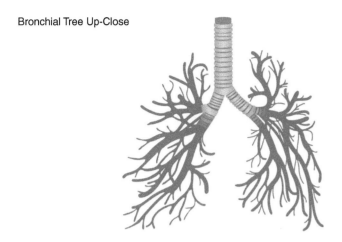

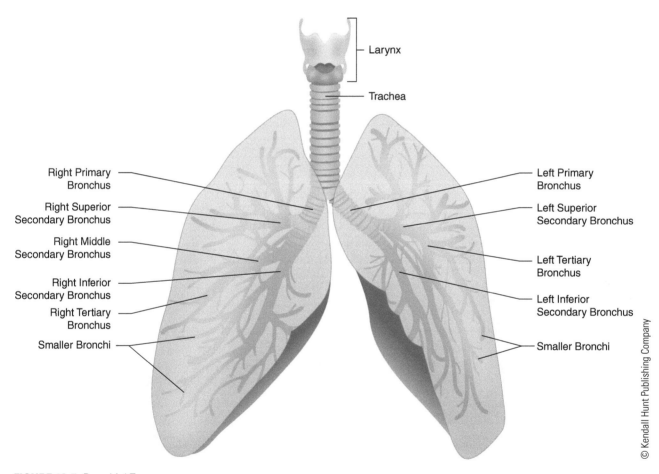

Larynx

Trachea

Right Primary Bronchus

Right Superior Secondary Bronchus

Right Middle Secondary Bronchus

Right Inferior Secondary Bronchus

Right Tertiary Bronchus

Smaller Bronchi

Left Primary Bronchus

Left Superior Secondary Bronchus

Left Tertiary Bronchus

Left Inferior Secondary Bronchus

Smaller Bronchi

© Kendall Hunt Publishing Company

FIGURE 19-5 Bronchial Tree

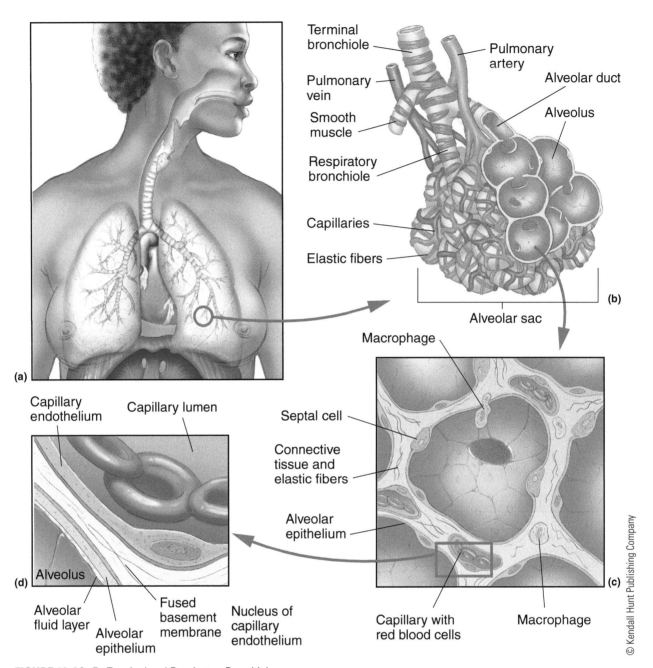

Terminal bronchiole
Pulmonary artery
Pulmonary vein
Alveolar duct
Smooth muscle
Alveolus
Respiratory bronchiole
Capillaries
Elastic fibers
Alveolar sac
Macrophage
Septal cell
Connective tissue and elastic fibers
Alveolar epithelium
Capillary with red blood cells
Macrophage
Capillary endothelium
Capillary lumen
Alveolus
Alveolar fluid layer
Alveolar epithelium
Fused basement membrane
Nucleus of capillary endothelium

(a) (b) (c) (d)

FIGURE 19-6A–D Terminal and Respiratory Bronchioles

IV. Lab Activity 19-1: Label these Structures

For BOTH Figs 19.7 & 19.8 below: MATCH the Listed Numbers with the Corresponding Letters on the Model Structures.

1. EPIGLOTTIS
2. VESTIBULAR FOLD/FALSE VOCAL CORD
3. TRUE VOCAL CORD
4. TRACHAE
5. THYROID CARTILAGE
6. CRICOTHYROID MEMBRANE
7. CRICOID CARTILAGE
8. GLOTTIS (OPENING)
9. CUNEIFORM CARTILAGE
10. EUSTACHIAN TUBE OPENING
11. HYOID BONE
12. THYROHYOID MEMBRANE
13. THYROID GLAND
14. ESOPHAGUS
15. HARD PALATE
16. LARYNGOPHARYNX
17. ORALPHARYNX
18. NASOPHARYNX
19. PALATE
20. PALATINE TONSILS
21. PHARYNGEAL TONSILS

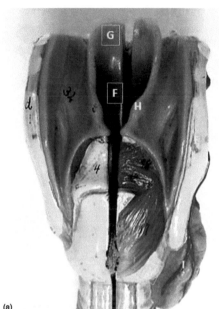

(a)

Item No. 1000272 [G21] - Larynx Model, 2 times full-size, © 3B Scientific GmbH, Germany, 2018, www.3bscientific.com. Photo by Pius Aboloye, MD.

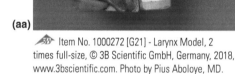

(aa)

Item No. 1000272 [G21] - Larynx Model, 2 times full-size, © 3B Scientific GmbH, Germany, 2018, www.3bscientific.com. Photo by Pius Aboloye, MD.

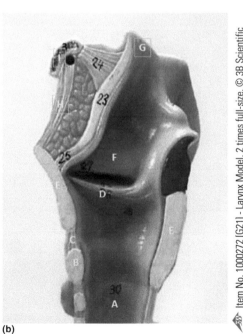

(b)

Item No. 1000272 [G21] - Larynx Model, 2 times full-size, © 3B Scientific GmbH, Germany, 2018, www.3bscientific.com. Photo by Pius Aboloye, MD.

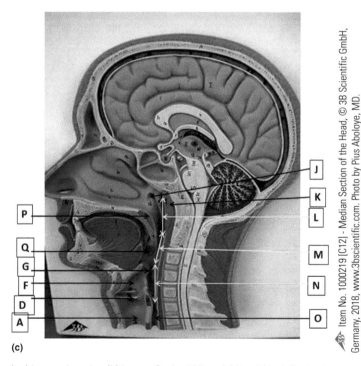

(c)

Item No. 1000219 [C12] - Median Section of the Head, © 3B Scientific GmbH, Germany, 2018, www.3bscientific.com. Photo by Pius Aboloye, MD.

FIGURE 19-7 Upper Respiratory Tract. (a) Larynx Posterior, (aa) Larynx Anterior, (b) Larynx Sagittal View, (c) Head-Neck Sagittal

1. UPPER LOBE
2. HORIZONTAL FISSURE
3. R. & L. OBLIQUE FISSURES
4. R. LOWER LOBE
5. L. PRIMARY BRONCHUS
6. R. SECONDARY (LOBAR) BRONCHUS
7. CARINA
8. L. TERTIARY BRONCHII
9. THORACIC AORTA
10. CARDIAC NOTCH
11. ESOPHAGUS
12. DIAPHRAGM
13. TRACHAE

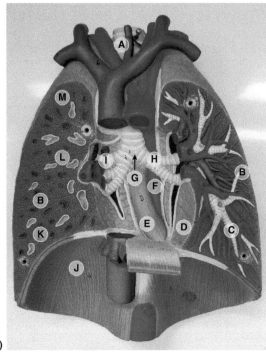

(a)

Item No. 1000270 [G15] - Lung model with larynx, © 3B Scientific GmbH, Germany, 2018, www.3bscientific.com. Photo by Pius Aboloye, MD.

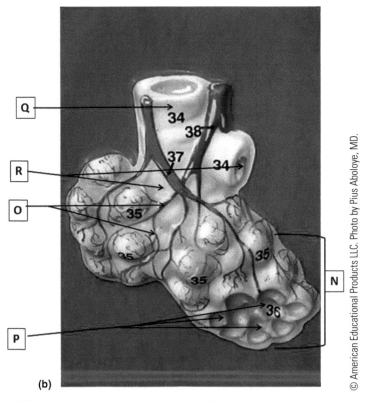

(b)

© American Educational Products LLC. Photo by Pius Aboloye, MD.

FIGURE 19-8 Thoracic Cavity and Alveolar Sac

V. Blood Circulation to the Lungs: Dual supply

A. **PULMONARY CIRCULATION:** Pulmonary trunk (artery) brings deoxygenated blood from right ventricle to the lungs. Pulmonary veins return oxygenated blood (from lung) to the left side of the left atrium.

B. **SYSTEMIC DISTRIBUTION:** Systemic (oxygenated) blood supply to the lungs is via the **bronchial arteries,** branches of the thoracic aorta.

Bronchial veins drain into the azygos and hemiazygos veins.

VI. Nerve Supply

A. **TO THE LUNGS: via pulmonary plexus of the vagus nerve.**

B. **TO THE DIAPHRAGM: via the phrenic nerve.**

VII. Muscles of Respiration

TABLE 19-4 Muscles of Respiration

MUSCLE	FUNCTION/ACTION WHEN CONTRACTED	EFFECT ON THORACIC DIMENSION (VOLUME)
INSPIRATION		
DIAPHRAGM	Primary muscle of inspiration (quite breathing). Flattens from its normal dome-shaped state.	Increases longitudinal diameter (volume).
EXTERNAL INTERCOASTAL	Second muscle of quiet breathing. Pulls the rib cage up and forward.	Increases anterior–posterior diameter (volume).
DEEP INSPIRATION		
EXTERNAL INTERCOASTAL	Pulls the rib cage up and forward.	Increases diameter (volume).
PECTORALIS MINOR	Pulls ribs 3, 4, 5 up, synergistic with external intercostal muscles and diaphragm.	Increases diameter (volume).
SCALENES	Pulls ribs 1, 2, 3 up, synergistic with external intercostal muscles and diaphragm.	Increases diameter (volume).
STERNOCLEIDOMASTOID	Pulls the sternum up, synergistic with external intercostal muscles and diaphragm.	Increases diameter (volume)
FORCED EXPIRATION		
INTERNAL INTERCOASTAL	Retracts and pull the rib cage down and back to normal.	Decreases anterior-posterior diameter (volume).
EXTERNAL OBLIQUE		
RECTUS ABDOMINIS	Compress the abdominal content, increases abdominal pressure and forces diaphragm superiorly, hence forcing air out of lungs.	Decreases longitudinal diameter (volume).

VIII. Clinical Applications in Respiratory System

TABLE 19-5 Clinical Applications in Respiratory System

TERMS/CONDITIONS	FEATURES
SINUSITIS	Inflammation of the mucosa lining of the sinuses resulting in increased pressure, pain, and headaches.
ENDOTRACHEAL INTUBATION	Procedure of inserting a flexible (ET) tube through the glottis and into trachea to provide airways for effective artificial ventilation using a laryngoscope to visualize the intubation/placement of the tube.
ASPIRATION PNEUMONIA	An inflammation of the lungs when foreign (food, etc.) are inhaled. Regurgitated food (from stomach) into the airways. Commonly in the elderly/people unable to protect airways.
ASTHMA	1 of 3 COPD patterned diseases. Inflammation of smaller airway bronchioles resulting in increased edema, mucus, narrowed lumen (bronchoconstriction), hence there's ventilation.
RESPIRATORY TRACT INFECTION	May be upper respiratory infection (URI) or lower respiratory infection (LRI) URI: from sinusitis to laryngitis, coughing is common. LRI: usually involves lower lung structures, as in bronchitis, pneumonia.
PNEUMOTHORAX	A collapsed lung. Negative pressure (partial vacuum) is required to fully inflate the alveoli. Increased air pressure in the pleura space, results in inability of the alveoli to fully expand and collapse. Causes: spontaneous lung rupture/penetrating thoracic wounds. Treatment is placement of chest tube with suctioning away of the air pressure from the space.
ATELECTASIS	Another type of collapsed lung but due to non-ventilation of alveoli (as in no deep breaths due to pain) seen in postoperative patients.
HICCUPS	Spasmodic contractions of diaphragm followed by the closure of the glottis resulting in the "hiccups" sounds. Normally harmless, but could be due CNS damage or nerve irritation.
COUGH	A protective reflex, caused by irritation of the trachea/bronchi.
SNEEZE	A protective reflex, caused by irritation of the nasal passage.
CHRONIC OBSTRUCTIVE PULMONARY DISEASE	COPD includes 3 chronic lung diseases: bronchitis, emphysema, and asthma.
TRACHEOTOMY	Surgical opening (and removal of part) of the trachea rings to provide airways for effective artificial ventilation.
CRICO-THYROIDOSTOMY	Emergent opening of the crico-thyroid membrane, usually done with a large needle) to provide for emergent effective artificial ventilation.
PLEURITIS	Aka pleurisy. Extremely painful inflammation of the pleura membrane especially with each breath taken.
CYSTIC FIBROSIS (CF)	Inherited disease of the exocrine glands resulting in thick mucus production which blocks ducts. Lungs, digestive tract, and sweat glands are often affected. Complications of CF include lung obstruction and collapse, recurrent lung infections, dehydration, and infertility (males).

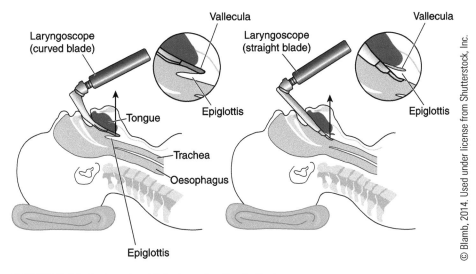

FIGURE 19-9A Endotracheal Tube Insertion (Intubation)

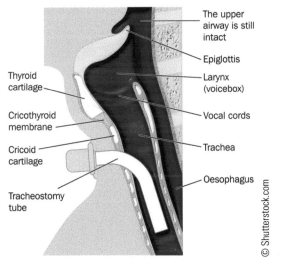

FIGURE 19-9B

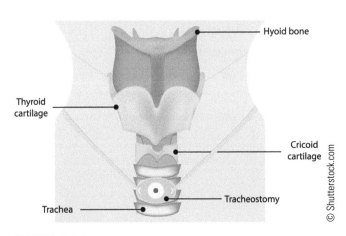

FIGURE 19-9C

IX. Lab Activity 19-2: Identify the Following Terms on the Models

A. LIST OF TERMINOLOGY: RESPIRATORY SYSTEM
(Use Figs: 19-7 & 19-8)

Lab Activity 19-2: Respiratory System

Identify the following Respiratory Structures on the Models

TERMINOLOGY LIST

- nasal cavity
- hard palate
- pharynx

- nasopharynx
- oropharynx
- laryngopharynx

- pharyngeal/palatine/lingual tonsils
- larynx
- epiglottis
- glottis
- thyroid cartilage
- cricoid cartilage
- cricothyroid membrane
- vestibular folds
- vocal folds
- thyroid gland
- trachea

- primary bronchus
- carina
- lobar (secondary) bronchus
- segmental (tertiary) bronchus
- lungs lobes
- fissures: oblique and transverse
- diaphragm
- external intercostal muscles
- internal intercostal muscles
- pectoralis minor muscle

B. **Answer the following questions:**

1. This portion of the pharynx receives both air and food:

   A. nasopharynx

   B. oropharynx

   C. laryngopharynx

   D. none of these

2. The vocal cords are located within the

   A. nasopharynx

   B. oropharynx

   C. larynx

   D. trachea

3. The larynx contains how many cartilages?

   A. 3

   B. 12

   C. 9

   D. 6

4. The last cartilage of the trachea as it divides into the right and left primary bronchus is also referred to as

   A. terminal bronchus

   B. carina

   C. lobar bronchus

   D. bronchioles

5. The oblique fissure of the left lung separates

   A. middle and superior lobes

   B. inferior and superior lobes

   C. middle and inferior lobes

   D. none of these

6. What are the components of the following?

   i) upper respiratory system

   ii) lower respiratory system

7. Compare and contrast emphysema and chronic bronchitis.

Digestive System

Upon completion of this exercise, you should be able to:

A. Describe the major functions of the digestive system.
B. Describe the histological structure of each of the four layers of the gastrointestinal (GI) wall: mucosa, submucosa, muscularis externa, and serosa (visceral peritoneum).
C. Define mastication and explain the importance in the overall digestive process.
D. Identify regions of the pharynx (naso-, oro-, and laryngopharynx) and classify the passage of food and/or air through them.
D. **Stomach:** List the regional parts and functions of stomach. Identify histological cells of the stomach and secretions of the cell types. Compare the muscle layers of stomach with those of small intestine.
E. **Small intestine (SI) and accessory organs:** List the different segments and functions of the SI. Describe the gross and histological features of the liver and pancreas with their secretions and functions. Describe in detail the bile flow from liver to duodenum.
E. **Large intestine (LI):** List the different segments of the colon, cecum, appendix, ileocecal valve, rectum, and anal sphincters.
F. List the blood supply and nerve supply to the different segments of the GI tract.
G. List the clinical applications.

NEEDED MATERIALS

1. Human torso: thorax and abdomen.
2. Models: stomach, duodenum/pancreas/liver/SI and LI.
3. Sagittal (median) head-neck model.
4. GI Wall plaque.
5. Microscope slides:
   - Esophagus
   - Stomach
   - SI
   - LI
   - Liver
   - Pancreas

Introduction

I. OVERVIEW

A. The digestive system includes the primary organ: alimentary canal or GI tract plus several accessory organs/structures (salivary gland, liver, gallbladder, and pancreas). This long continuous GI tube has several regions with different functions, including the esophagus, stomach, SI, and LI.

B.

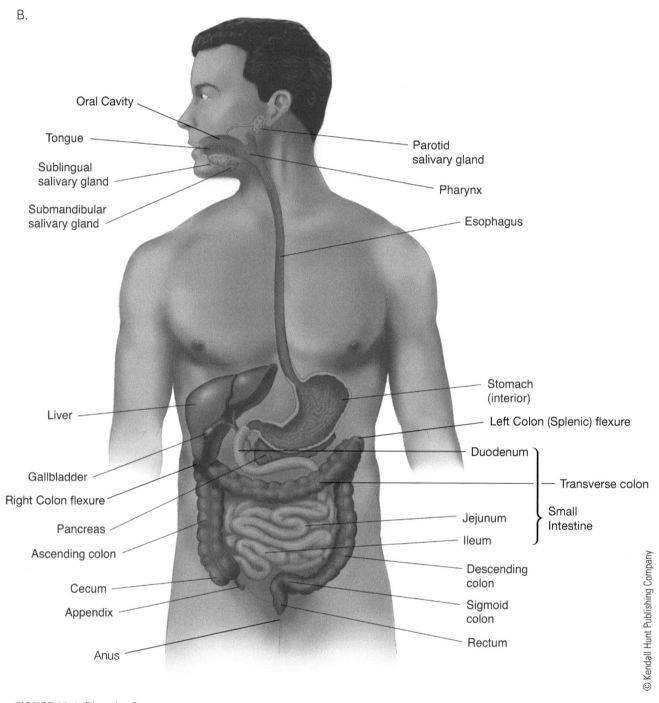

FIGURE 20-1 Digestive System

C. The digestive system performs multiple functions, including but not limited to the following:
   Seven steps/processes are involved in the digestion and absorption of nutrients:

   1. Ingestion: putting the food in the mouth.
   2. Mastication: chewing to increase the surface area for enzyme action.
   3. Deglutition: the act of swallowing.
   4. Secretion of enzymes, bile, acid, water, and mucus.
   5. Digestion: Both mechanical (churning) and chemical (enzyme) breakdown of food materials.

6. Absorption: Transfer of the products of digestion from GI lumen into blood or lacteal.

7. Defecation: The act of removing undigested/unabsorbed food materials from the body via the rectum.

D. **PERITONEUM:** The serous membrane of the abdomen has two layers: outer parietal and inner visceral (on the organ). The peritoneal cavity is the potential cavity between these two layers of peritoneum.

   The peritoneum has several folds which are continuous (but with different names), as it wraps around GI structures.

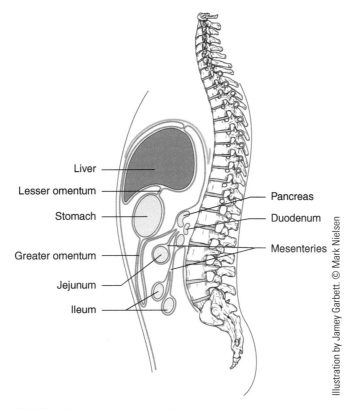

FIGURE 20-2 Mesentaries and Omenta

Peritoneum Folds:

1. Greater omentum, the double layer of peritoneum, hangs from the greater curvature of the stomach and then drapes over the transverse colon and in front of all abdominal organs.

2. Lesser omentum is the peritoneal fold from the lesser curvature of the stomach to the anterior–inferior edge of the liver. Hepatic portal vein, hepatic artery, and vagus nerve travel in this structure.

3. Falciform ligament connects the liver to the diaphragm and the anterior abdominal wall.

4. Mesentery proper attaches the jejunum and the ileum to the posterior body wall.

5. Mesocolon suspends the different parts of the colon to the posterior wall.

6. **Peritoneal versus retroperitoneal organs:** Not all GI structures are enclosed within the peritoneum membrane. Organs that are behind this massive wrap of peritoneum are called retroperitoneal organs (e.g., duodenum, pancreas, kidneys, bladder, aorta, inferior vena cava, sigmoid colon, rectum). All other organs within the cavity are referred to as peritoneal organs.

E. GROSS ANATOMY OF THE GI TRACT: Layers of the alimentary canal

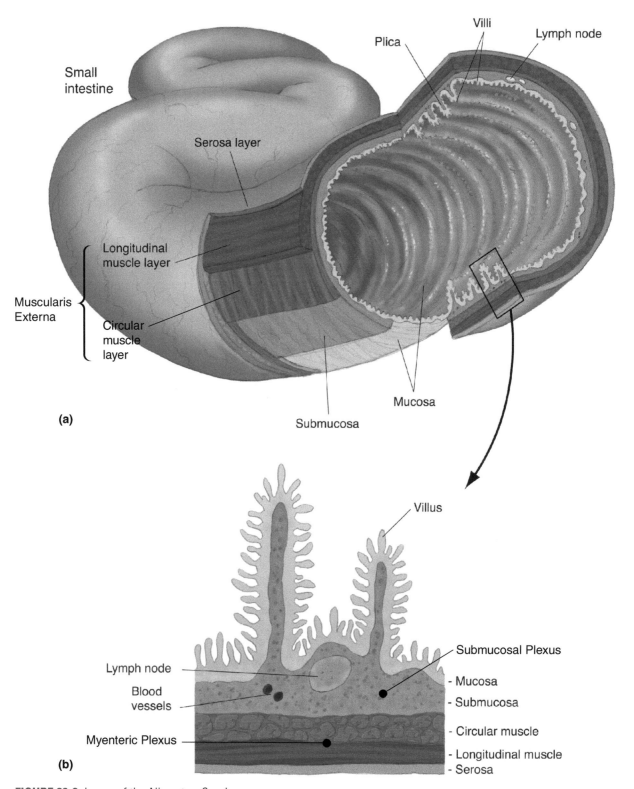

FIGURE 20-3 Layers of the Alimentary Canal

TABLE 20-1 Layers of the GI Tract

LAYER	STRUCTURE	DESCRIPTION
Mucosa	Epithelium	Subtype changes throughout the GI tract.
	Lamina Propria	Areolar connective tissue that attaches epithelium to the muscularis mucosae. Contains MALT in some locations.
	Muscularis Mucosae	Thin layer of smooth muscle that creates folds in the stomach and small intestine, increasing surface area.
Submucosa		Areolar connective tissue that connects the mucosa to the muscularis externa. Contains blood vessels, lymphatics, and an extensive network of neurons called the *submucosal plexus*.
Muscularis Externa	Circular Muscle	Inner layer of smooth muscle; contributes to the mixing movements and *peristalsis* in the GI tract; *myenteric plexus* located between circular and longitudinal layers.
	Longitudinal Muscle	Outer layer of smooth muscle; contributes to the mixing movements and *peristalsis* in the GI tract; *myenteric plexus* located between circular and longitudinal layers.
Serosa		Serous membrane that is the superficial layer found on portions of the GI tract in the abdominopelvic cavity; *adventitia* composed of areolar connective tissue and exposed collagen fibers on portions of the GI tract outside the abdominopelvic cavity.

F.

TABLE 20-2 Movement Types of the GI Tract

MOVEMENT	FEATURES AND LOCATION WHERE COMMONLY FOUND
CHURNING	Mechanical mixing of food, enzymes, and acids. It is specific to the stomach, and its function is to increase digestion by digestive enzymes.
PERISTALSIS	A rhythmic, wave-like movement that progressively moves materials (forward) through a hollow tubular organ (e.g., small intestine, ureters, fallopian tube). Peristalsis takes place throughout the entire GI tract.
SEGMENTATION	Is defined as alternating contractions allowing for regional mixing of intestinal contents back and forth. Common to the small intestine.
MASS MOVEMENT	Also referred to as "giant migrating contractions." A series of waves together that is like an intense but prolonged peristalsis contraction, often resulting in evacuation of the colonic content. Localized to the colon only.

II. Mouth to Esophagus

A.

TABLE 20-3 Mouth to Esophagus: Structures

MAJOR STRUCTURES	FEATURES AND FUNCTIONS
TONGUE	Primary organ used for taste, has several projections (papilla) and taste buds. Is a thick skeletal muscle structure. Also used for mastication, deglutition, and speech.
PAPILLAE	3 types: **1. Vallate:** The largest but only 8–10 in number, divides the tongue into an anterior two-third and a posterior one-third. They have taste buds in them. **2. Fungiform:** Second largest and numerous, also has taste buds. **3. Filiform:** The smallest and most numerous. Have no taste buds.
TEETH	An accessory organ. Primarily for mastication of food into smaller particles. 2 types: 1. Desiduous/milk: Appears after 6 months of age, but later sheds. 2. Permanent: Appears later. Consists of incisors, canine, premolars, and molars. The crown is made of dentin (cellular active below) and is covered by the enamel (acellular inactive, toughest structure in human body).
SALIVARY GLANDS	An accessory organ of digestion. Produce salivary amylase that aids in the digestion of carbohydrates. **1. Parotid gland, 2. Submandibular gland, and 3. Sublingual gland.**
PALATE	Hard palate forms the roof of the mouth, separates the nasal and oral cavities. Soft palate is found on the posterior edge of the hard palate, mostly mucous membrane, soft tissues, and glands. Uvula and palatine tonsils can be found in the soft palate.
PHARYNX	A tubular structure located posteriorly on the pharyngeal wall from below the occipital bone down the level of the larynx. Has 3 parts: **1. Nasopharynx** (respiratory function only), **2. Oropharynx** (respiratory and digestive), and **3. Laryngopharynx** (respiratory and digestive).
ESOPHAGUS	Conduct food from the oropharynx into the stomach. Upper two-third is skeletal muscle, lower one-third is smooth muscle. The thorax part travels behind the heart and enters the abdomen via the esophageal hiatus (opening) in the diaphragm. The esophagus has adventitia instead of a true serosa covering.
GASTROESOPHAGEAL (GE) JUNCTION	The abdominal portion of the esophagus is short, meets the stomach at the (transition) GE junction. The GE sphincter is located inside here.
GASTROESOPHAGEAL (GE) OR CARDIAC SPHINCTER	Opening of the distal (abdominal portion) esophagus into the stomach. A physiologic sphincter that prevents reflux/regurgitation into the esophagus.

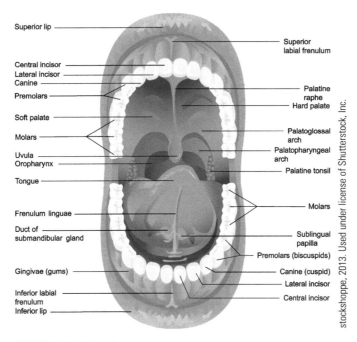

FIGURE 20-4 Mouth

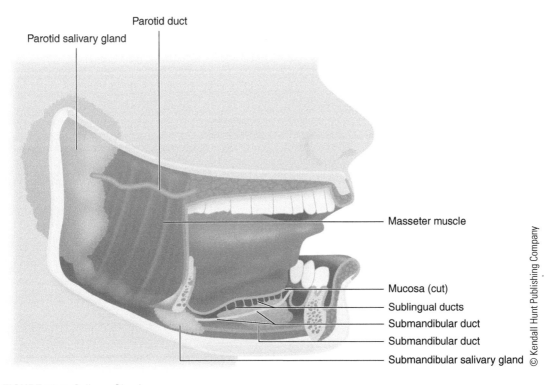

FIGURE 20-5 Salivary Glands

B. **PHARYNX PARTS AND FUNCTION:** Nasopharynx (allows for air passage only), oropharynx, and laryngopharynx (the last two allow for both air and food passage). The laryngopharynx is continuous with esophagus.

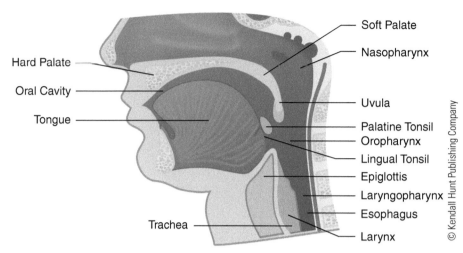

FIGURE 20-6 Pharynx

C. MUSCLES OF MASTICATION: The act of chewing functions to break down the food into smaaller particles, increasing surface area for digestive enzymes' activity. They include the masseter, temporalis, buccinators, and the pterygoid (lateral and medial) muscles.

D. TEETH

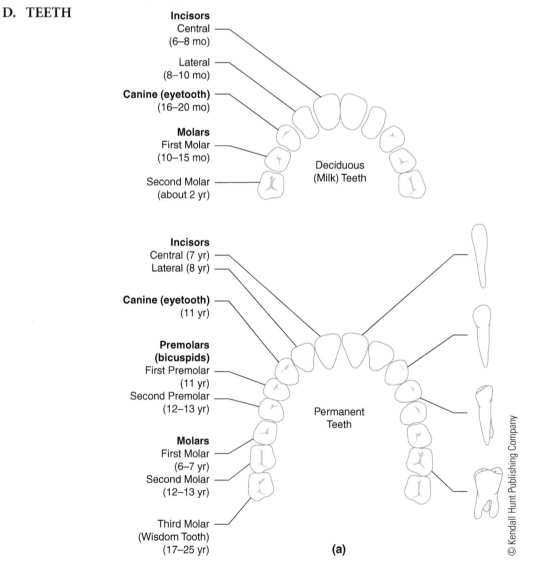

FIGURE 20-7A Tooth Structure

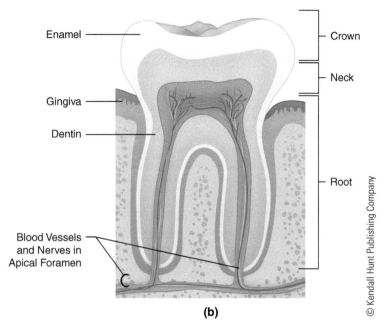

Enamel

Crown

Neck

Gingiva

Dentin

Root

Blood Vessels
and Nerves in
Apical Foramen

© Kendall Hunt Publishing Company

(b)

FIGURE 20-7B Tooth Structure (*continued*)

III. Stomach

A

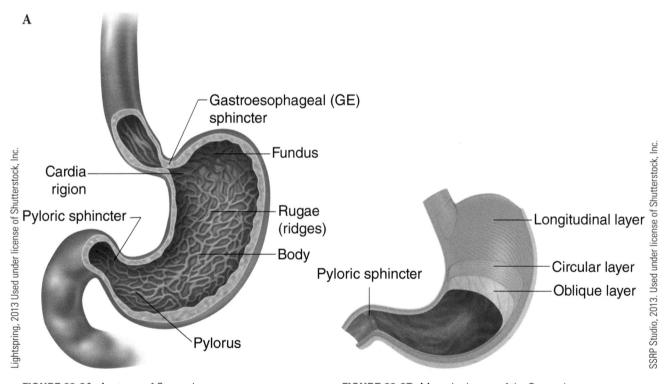

Gastroesophageal (GE)
sphincter

Fundus

Cardia
rigion

Rugae
(ridges)

Pyloric sphincter

Body

Pylorus

Lightspring, 2013 Used under license of Shutterstock, Inc.

Pyloric sphincter

Longitudinal layer

Circular layer

Oblique layer

SSRP Studio, 2013. Used under license of Shutterstock, Inc.

FIGURE 20-8A Anatomy of Stomach

FIGURE 20-8B Muscular Layers of the Stomach

B

TABLE 20-4 Stomach Structures

MAJOR STRUCTURES	FEATURES AND FUNCTIONS
CARDIAC REGION	Between the abdominal portion of the esophagus and the stomach. Gastroesophageal (GE) junction where the 2 meet. Is part of this cardiac area. GE (muscle) sphincter is located inside region.
GE SPHINCTER	Opening of the distal esophagus into the stomach. A physiologic sphincter that prevents reflux/regurgitation into the esophagus.
FUNDUS	The superior dome-shaped portion lies to the left of the cardiac region.
BODY	The area just below the cardiac and fundus but not including the pylorus. Largest region.
RUGAE	Mucosa folds of the stomach, allows for increased surface area.
PYLORUS (CANAL) REGION	The tubular distal portion of the stomach as it joins with the duodenum. The pyloric sphincter is located within.
PYLORUS SPHINCTER	The thick muscular wall of pylorus where the stomach opens into the duodenum. It is both an anatomical and a physiological sphincter that controls the rate of stomach content emptying into the duodenum.
GREATER CURVATURE	Left side border (convex) of the stomach, the greater omentum attaches here and drapes inferiorly over the transverse colon. The gastrosplenic ligament attaches the stomach to spleen at the far left of the curvature.
LESSER CURVATURE	Right side border (concave) of the stomach, the lesser omentum (hepatogastric ligament) attaches here. Gastric vessels and the hepatic portal vein travel in this.
MUCOSA CELL TYPES OF THE GASTRIC PIT	
■ MUCUS NECK CELLS	Produces alkaline mucus, to prevent self-digestion.
■ PARIETAL CELLS	Secretes hydrochloric acid (HCl) and intrinsic factor. Intrinsic factor is necessary for vitamin B12 absorption (occurs in terminal ileum). HCl is important in the conversion of pepsinogen (inactive) to pepsin (active) enzyme for protein digestion.
■ CHIEF CELLS	Produces pepsinogen (inactive), which is then converted by HCl (parietal cell) into active pepsin. Pepsin begins protein digestion in the stomach.
■ ENTERO-ENDOCRINE GLANDS	Found deepest in the pit, secretes gastric hormones (gastrin, histamine, and somatostatin), which regulate gastric digestion.

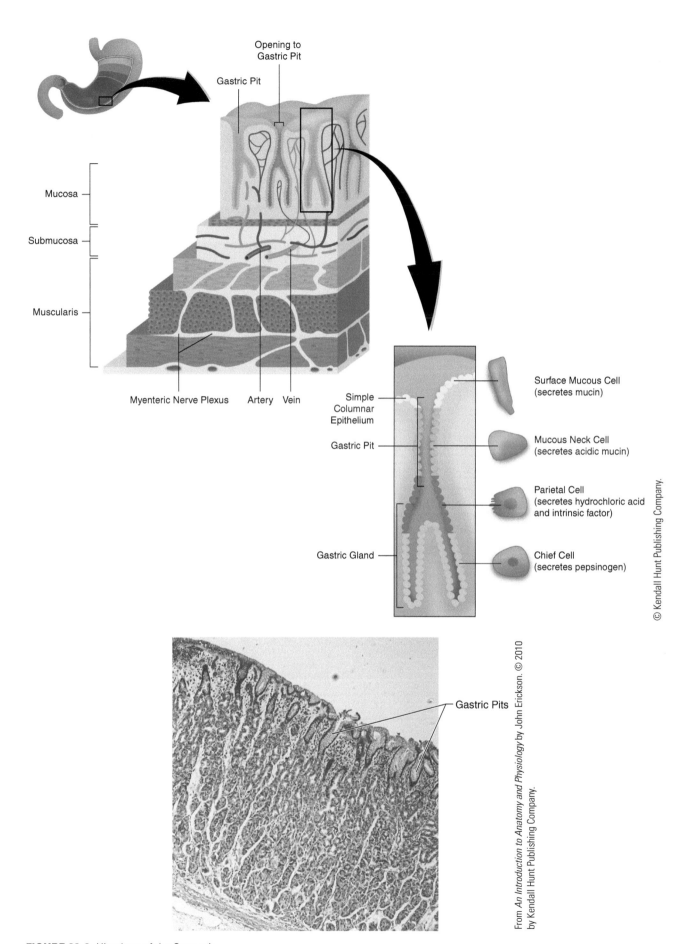

Opening to
Gastric Pit

Gastric Pit

Mucosa

Submucosa

Muscularis

Myenteric Nerve Plexus   Artery   Vein

Simple
Columnar
Epithelium

Gastric Pit

Gastric Gland

Surface Mucous Cell
(secretes mucin)

Mucous Neck Cell
(secretes acidic mucin)

Parietal Cell
(secretes hydrochloric acid
and intrinsic factor)

Chief Cell
(secretes pepsinogen)

© Kendall Hunt Publishing Company.

Gastric Pits

From *An Introduction to Anatomy and Physiology* by John Erickson. © 2010
by Kendall Hunt Publishing Company.

FIGURE 20-9 Histology of the Stomach

C. BLOOD SUPPLY:

i) **Arteries:** Blood supply to the stomach and upper GI structures comes from branches of the **celiac** artery (the first major branch of the abdominal aorta). Left and right gastric arteries supply the lesser curvature, and the gastroepiploic arteries supply the greater curvature.

ii) **Veins:** Left and right gastric veins drain into the hepatic portal vein.

iii) **Nerve supply** has both sympathetic and parasympathetic (via vagus) innervations.

IV. Small Intestine and Accessory Organs

A

TABLE 20-5 Small Intestine Structures

MAJOR STRUCTURES	FEATURES AND FUNCTIONS
DUODENUM	A C-shaped tube, curves around the head of the pancreas. Shortest part of the SI about 10 in. long. First part (top of the C): receives stomach chyme via the pyloric sphincter. Second part (middle of the C): major pancreatic ducts and common bile ducts open into the duodenum via the duodenal papilla here. Third part (bottom of the C): forms a flexure that is continuous with the jejunum.
JEJUNUM	Second part of the SI and is ~8 ft. long. Most digestion and absorption of nutrients takes place in the jejunum and ileum.
ILEUM	Third part of SI and is ~12 ft. long. Most digestion and absorption of nutrients takes place in the jejunum and ileum.
ILEOCECAL VALVE	A functional sphincter that controls the flow of contents (undigested food) from ileum into cecum.
PLICA CIRCULARIS	Permanent mucosal folds of the SI wall, allows for increased surface area for absorption.
PEYER PATCHES	Mucosal lymphatic tissues of the SI, for immunity. Abundant in the ileum.

B

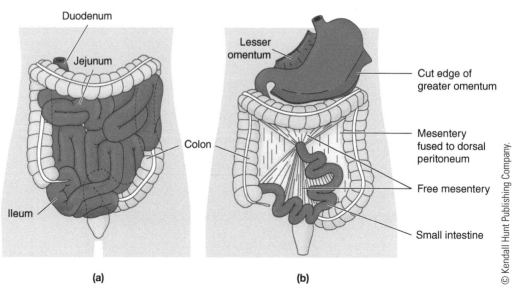

FIGURE 20-10 Anatomy of Small Intestine

© Kendall Hunt Publishing Company.

DIGESTIVE SYSTEM

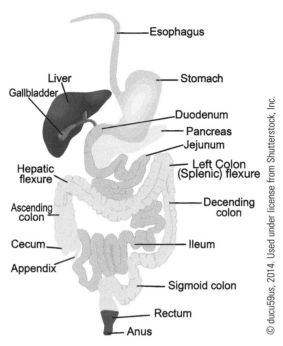

FIGURE 20-11 Anatomy of Small Intestine

C

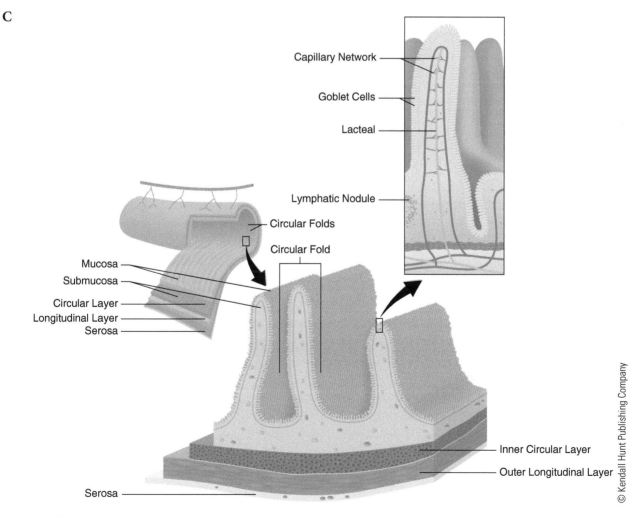

FIGURE 20-12 Small Intestine Folds

D

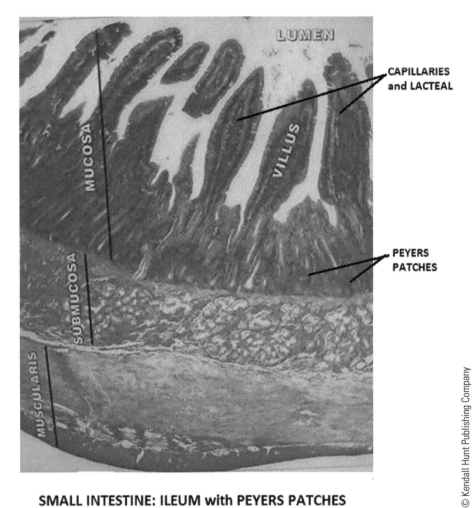

SMALL INTESTINE: ILEUM with PEYERS PATCHES

FIGURE 20-13 Histology Slide Ileum

E. **ACCESORY ORGANS AND GLANDS:**
   I)

TABLE 20-6 Accessory Organs and Glands

MAJOR STRUCTURES	FEATURES AND FUNCTIONS
SALIVARY GLANDS	Produce salivary amylase that aids in the digestion of carbohydrates. **1. Parotid gland, 2. Submandibular gland, and 3. Sublingual gland.**
EXOCRINE PANCREAS	The organ has 3 major parts: head-neck, body, and tail. Acini cells: digestive enzymes for carbohydrate, protein, and fat digestion.
ENDOCRINE PANCREAS	Pancreatic islets (of Langerhans), consist of alpha cells (glucagon secretion) and beta cells (insulin secretion).
LIVER	Largest organ in the human body, located below the diaphragm. It has a large right lobe (further subdivided into quadrate and caudate lobes by the gall bladder and IVC) and a smaller left lobe. Several functions: bile production, storage of nutrients, detoxification, and production of plasma proteins among others.
GALL BLADDER	Located on the undersurface of the liver. Primary function is to store and concentrate bile (produced by the liver).

MAJOR STRUCTURES	FEATURES AND FUNCTIONS
DUCT SYSTEM	1. **Cystic duct:** from the gallbladder joins the common hepatic duct to form common bile duct. 2. **Common hepatic duct:** formed by the union of the right and left hepatic ducts. 3. **Common bile duct:** formed by the joining of the common hepatic and cystic ducts. Descends inferiorly and travels posteriorly through the head of the pancreas before joining with **main pancreatic duct. Both of** the ducts then have same opening into the duodenum at the duodenal papilla.

II)

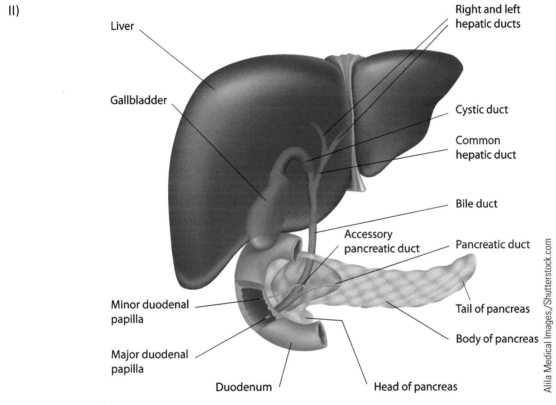

FIGURE 20-14A Liver/Gallbladder/Pancreas/Duodenum

III)

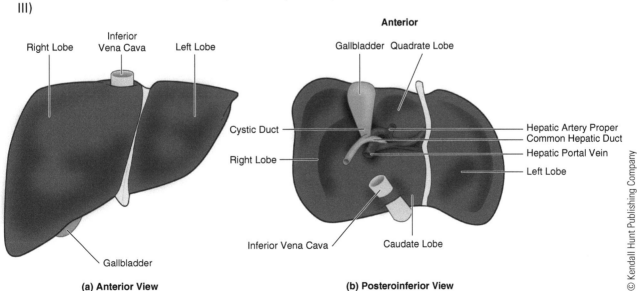

(a) Anterior View   **(b) Posteroinferior View**

FIGURE 20-14B Liver Anatomy

F. HISTOLOGY SLIDES: PANCREAS & LIVER:

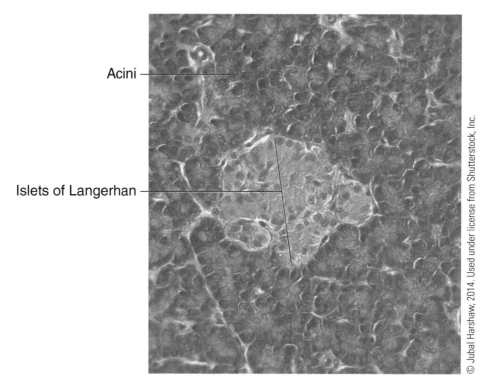

Acini

Islets of Langerhan

FIGURE 20-15 Pancreas

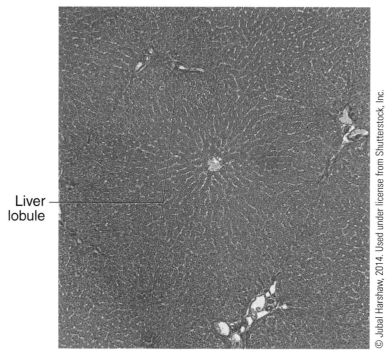

Liver
lobule

FIGURE 20-16 Liver

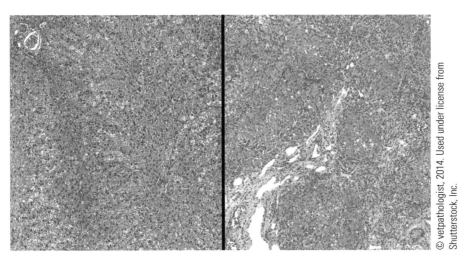

© vetpathologist, 2014. Used under license from Shutterstock, Inc.

FIGURE 20-17 Normal Liver (left) vs. Abnormal Liver (Right) compared

G. BLOOD SUPPLY:

i) **Arteries:** Blood supply to the jejunum, ileum, and about two-third of the colon (to the splenic flexure) comes from branches of the superior mesentery artery (the second major branch of the abdominal aorta). These branches anastomose to form arcades.

ii) **Veins:** The veins drain into superior mesentery vein, which eventually drains into the hepatic portal vein.

iii) **Nerve supply:** Both sympathetic and parasympathetic (via vagus) innervations form the superior mesentery plexus.

V. Large Intestine

A.

TABLE 20-7 Large Intestinal Structures

MAJOR STRUCTURES	FEATURES AND FUNCTIONS
CECUM	First part of the colon; a blind pouch located in the iliac fossa. Has the appendix on the posterior-medial aspect. Receives undigested food from the terminal ileum through the ileocecal valve, continues as the ascending colon.
APPENDIX	Located on the posterior-medial wall of the cecum, is a narrow tube which a remnants of the celom
COLON	Also known as large intestine. Segments include: cecum, ascending colon, right colon (hepatic) flexure, transverse, left colon (splenic) flexure, descending, sigmoid, rectum, and anal canal.
HAUSTRUM	These are sacculations (haustra) formed by the taeniae coli bands.
EPIPLOIC (OMENTAL) APPENDAGES	Small fatty (folds) of peritoneum attached to the colon exterior often along the taeniae.
TAENIA COLI	3 bands of longitudinal smooth muscle on the exterior of the colon, forms the haustra.
RECTUM	The last 15 cm of the colon and is continuous with the anal canal. Functions primarily as a storage site, until emptied by defecation.
ANAL CANAL	A short segment tube. Has 2 sphincters, both must relax/open to be able to defecate. **Internal sphincter:** made up of smooth muscles and under autonomic nervous control. **External sphincter:** made up of skeletal muscles (of the pelvic diaphragm) and under conscious (voluntary) control.

B.

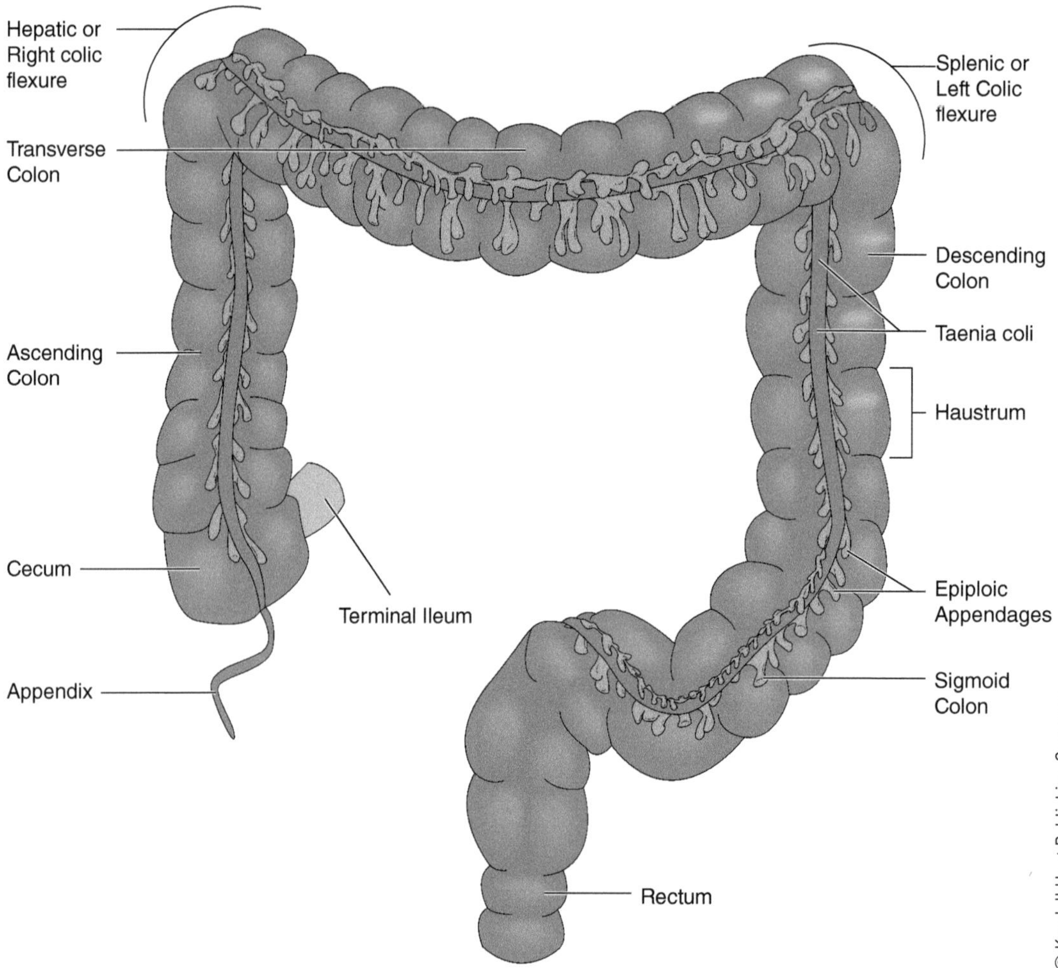

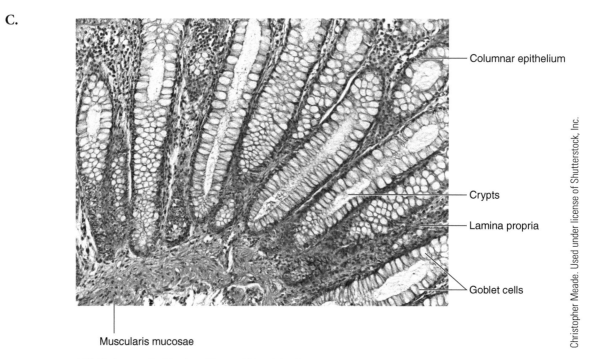

Hepatic or Right colic flexure

Transverse Colon

Ascending Colon

Cecum

Appendix

Terminal Ileum

Splenic or Left Colic flexure

Descending Colon

Taenia coli

Haustrum

Epiploic Appendages

Sigmoid Colon

Rectum

© Kendall Hunt Publishing Company

FIGURE 20-18A Anatomy of the Colon

C.

Columnar epithelium

Crypts

Lamina propria

Goblet cells

Muscularis mucosae

Christopher Meade. Used under license of Shutterstock, Inc.

FIGURE 20-18B Histology Tissue Slide of the Colon

VI. Blood Supply to the Large Intestine

i) **Arteries:** Blood supply to the cecum, and ascending and transverse colon up to the splenic flexure comes from branches of the **superior mesentery** artery (the second major branch of the abdominal aorta). These branches anastomose to form arcades. Descending and sigmoid colon supply is by the inferior mesentery artery.

ii) **Veins:** The veins drain into superior mesentery and inferior mesentery veins, which eventually drain into the hepatic portal vein.

iii) **Nerve supply:** Both sympathetic and parasympathetic (via vagus) innervations form the superior mesentery plexus and inferior hypogastric plexus.

VII. Nerve Supply

A. Nerve supply to the GI tract is dual via the vagus nerve plexus (parasympathetic) for digestion/secretion. Sympathetic innervation is via the splanchnic nerves.

VIII. Clinical Applications Digestive Diseases

A.

TABLE 20-8 Clinical Applications in Digestion System

TERMS/CONDITIONS	DIAGNOSTIC FEATURES
GASTRITIS	Inflammation of the gastric mucosa; causes: aspirin, alcohol, or infection. May present with stomach pain and hematemesis.
GASTROENTERITIS	Diffuse inflammation of the GI tract, stomach, and small intestine involvement. Symptoms of fever nausea/vomiting/diarrhea with abdominal discomfort. Food- and water-borne infection: bacteria, virus, or protozoa.
HIATAL HERNIA	Protrusion of the fundus of the stomach, into the thorax through a dilated esophageal opening (hiatus) in the diaphragm. Symptoms include indigestion, heartburn following meals, and acid reflux. Diagnosis is made via a Barium swallow study (X-ray) or CT scan.
PEPTIC ULCER	Erosion of the gastric (or duodenum) mucosa due to *Helicobacter pylori* (bacteria) infection and presence of high pepsin in the stomach. Presents with pain, GI bleeding. Diagnosis is via an upper GI endoscopy. *Treatment*: combination therapy of proton pump inhibitors, acid-reducing agents plus antibiotic.
HEPATITIS B	Blood-borne or sexually transmitted viral infection, presents with fever, jaundice, and enlarged tender liver. It is diagnosed following serum immunoglobulins for viral hepatitis B. May lead to chronic hepatitis and cirrhosis.
HEPATITIS C	Blood-borne or sexually transmitted viral infection, presents with fever and jaundice (enlarged tender liver). It is diagnosed following serum immunoglobulins for viral hepatitis C. May lead to chronic hepatitis and cirrhosis.
CIRRHOSIS	Liver damage secondary to alcohol or chronic hepatitis. Symptoms at presentation: jaundice, upper abdominal tenderness, ascites, bleeding tendencies, and hepatic coma in end-stage disease. Liver transplant or death.
CHOLECYSTITIS	Inflammation of the gallbladder due to infection or less commonly tumor. Presents with mid-epigastric abdominal pain following ingestion of greasy food, nausea, vomiting, and fever, may be jaundiced. Ultrasound is diagnostic tool of choice. Treatment is cholecystectomy.

TABLE 20-8 (*Continued*)

TERMS/CONDITIONS	DIAGNOSTIC FEATURES
CHOLELITHIASIS	A condition of gallstone presence in gallbladder, usually with no symptoms. If patient presents with fever, mid-epigastric pain, etc., then it is cholecystitis. Treatment is same as for cholecystitis: cholecystectomy.
COLOSTOMY	A surgical opening between the colon and skin, as in colon diversion. Often performed for colorectal cancer surgery removal.
PANCREATITIS	Inflammation of the pancreas, most common causes: alcohol and gallstones stuck in the common bile duct as it passes through the head of the pancreas. Acute abdominal pain, jaundice. Diagnosis: serum pancreatic enzymes and CT scan. Fluid and electrolyte replacement is treatment.
PANCREATIC CANCER	Mostly deadly cancer with low survival rate at 5 years. Linked to smoking, alcohol abuse, and chronic pancreatitis. Symptoms of malabsorption, jaundice, and upper abdominal pain. Diagnosis: CT scan and needle biopsy. Poor prognosis.
APPENDICITIS	Acute inflammation of the appendix secondary to fecal impaction of its lumen. Right lower quadrant abdominal pain, nausea/vomiting +/- fever. Treatment: Appendectomy.
DIVERTICULOSIS	Diverticula (out-pouching) of the colon wall due to increased intraluminal pressure from chronic constipation. Diverticulosis is a condition with no symptoms. In diverticulitis, the diverticuli are impacted with fecal material, and become inflamed, pain results. Colonoscopy is diagnostic tool of choice. Treatment: antibiotics plus recommended high-fiber diet and stool softener. If perforated, then colon resection is warranted.
CROHN DISEASE	An autoimmune inflammatory disease affecting both the small intestine and the colon. It is a transmural (all layers of the wall) disease skipping the segments of the GI. The scared/fibrotic walls lack absorptive ability. Symptoms of malabsorption, diarrhea, constipation, or hematochezia (bloody stool) are common with fever in the acute phase. Treatment: IV antibiotics, steroids, and fluids with bowel rest. Surgical resection of severely diseased segments may be warranted.
ULCERATIVE COLITIS	An autoimmune inflammatory disease affecting colon only. But the colon mucosa alone is involved. Symptoms of diarrhea, constipation, or hematochezia (bloody stool) are common with fever in the acute phase. Treatment: IV antibiotics, steroids, and fluids with bowel rest. Plus immune suppressant drugs.
COLORECTAL CANCER	No 3 most common and no 2 cause of cancer death in both men and women combined in the United States (2014). Risks factors: family history, previous cancer history, inflammatory bowel disease, adenomatous polyps, and smoking. Symptoms include changes in bowel movement and painless hematochezia (bloody stool). Screening includes routine rectal examination, sigmoidoscopy, and colonoscopy with biopsy. Treatment depends on the stage of the disease: surgical resection plus adjuvant chemo- and/or radiotherapy.
PERITONITIS	Inflammation of the peritoneum coverings secondary to an infection. Very serious complications include death or severe bowel adhesions, if patient survives.

IX. Lab Activity: Identify the Following Terms on the Models

A.

TABLE 20-9 List of Terminology in Digestive System

Mouth–Esophagus
- parotid glands
- submandibular glands
- sublingual glands
- esophagus
- gastroesophageal (GE) junction
- structural sphincter (GE Sphincter) valve

Stomach
- fundus
- body
- muscles: circular, longitudinal, oblique
- pylorus (antrium)
- lesser curvature
- greater curvature
- rugae
- pyloric sphincter

Small Intestine
- duodenum
- duodenal papilla
- sphincter of oddi
- jejunum: plica circulares
- ileum
- ileocecal sphincter (valve)

Large Intestine
- cecum
- appendix
- ascending colon, transverse, sigmoid colon
- hepatic and splenic flexure
- tinea coli
- haustra, epiploic appendages

- rectum
- internal and external anal sphincters
- pelvic (urogenital) diaphragm

Liver
- gall bladder
- hepatic duct
- cystic duct
- common bile duct

Pancreas
- pancreatic duct
- ampulla of Vater (hepatopancreatic ampulla)

- greater omentum
- lesser omentum
- mesentery
- spleen

Abdominal Vessels
- abdominal aorta
- celiac trunk
- splenic artery
- common hepatic artery
- hepatic artery
- superior mesenteric artery
- inferior mesenteric artery
- inferior vena cava vein
- hepatic portal vein (and its branches)
  - gastric veins
  - splenic vein
  - superior mesenteric vein
  - inferior mesenteric vein

GI Tissue Slides
- Stomach: gastric pits
- duodenum
- ileum: Peyers patches
- colon
- pancreas
- liver

X. Post-Lab Activity: Digestive System (Label these Structures)

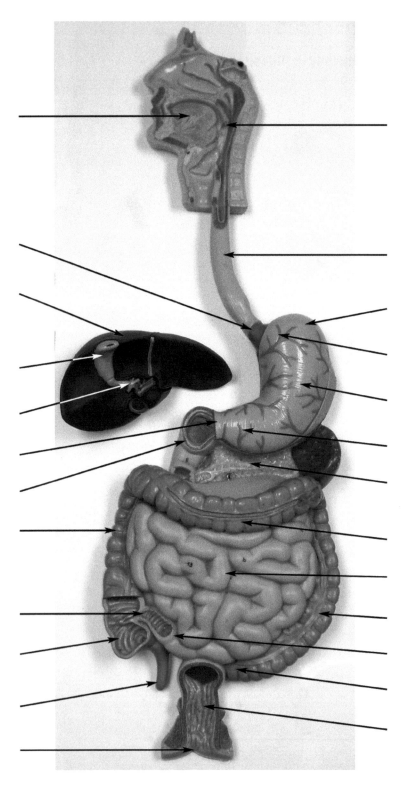

FIGURE 20-19 Digestive System Anatomy

Item No. 1000306 [K20] - Digestive System, © 3B Scientific GmbH, Germany, 2018, www.3bscientific.com. Photo by Pius Aboloye, MD.

Mucosa

Submucosa

Muscularis

Serosa

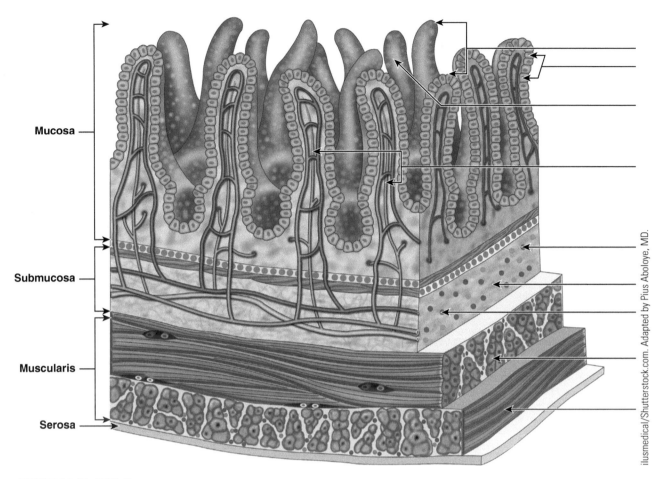

ilusmedical/Shutterstock.com. Adapted by Pius Aboloye, MD.

FIGURE 20-20 GI Wall

A. Identify these GI tissue slides:

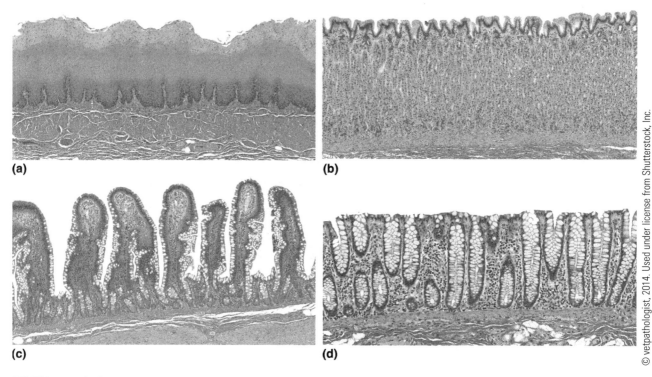

(a)　　　(b)　　　(c)　　　(d)

FIGURE 20-21A–D

B. Answer the following questions:

1. The taenia coli are

   A. three longitudinal bands of muscle located on the colon

   B. folds of mucosa in the colon

   C. outer pouches of the large intestine

   D. three longitudinal bands of muscle located on the stomach

2. Which of these listed structures is not considered part of the primary organ of digestive system?

   A. stomach

   B. spleen

   C. colon

   D. pharynx

3. The stomach has this additional layer of muscle:

   A. skeletal

   B. circular

   C. oblique

   D. longitudinal

4. Digestion of food begins in the

   A. mouth

   B. stomach

   C. duodenum

   D. jejunum

5. Most absorption of nutrients (post digestion) takes place in the
    A. cecum
    B. duodenum
    C. ileum
    D. jejunum

6. What are rugae and plicae circularis? List their function(s) and locations.

7. List the major regions of the colon.

8. Describe bile flow from the liver into the small intestine.

9. Distinguish between the exocrine and the endocrine pancreas.

10. Distinguish between diverticulosis and diverticulitis.

Urinary System

Upon completion of this exercise, you should be able to:

A. Describe the major functions of the urinary system.
B. Identify the gross and microscopic features of the kidneys.
C. List the parts of the nephron and their functions.
D. List the main blood vessels of the kidney.
E. Describe the steps in urine formation.
F. List the structures and functions of the ureters and urinary bladder.
G. Compare and contrast the male and female urethra.
H. List the clinical applications.

NEEDED MATERIALS

1. Human torso: abdomen and pelvis.
2. Models: kidney, nephron, and renal corpuscle.
3. Model: kidney, ureter, and bladder (KUB) stand.
4. Male reproductive organ (for urethra identification).
5. Pig kidney.
6. Dissection tray/instrument/gloves.
7. Microscope slide: kidney.

Introduction

I. OVERVIEW

A. The renal system includes theses organs: **paired kidneys, paired ureters, the cystic bladder (1), and the single urethra.**

Located high in the posterior abdominal cavity, the kidneys (as well as the bladder) are considered retroperitoneal organs. Atop both kidneys are the suprarenal/adrenal glands. The left kidney is slightly higher than the right, because of the position of the large right lobe liver on the right side.

The two kidneys form urine by filtering blood plasma. After several steps, the formed urine flows from kidneys into the ureters by gravity (and peristalsis) into the urinary/cystic bladder where it is stored until ready to be excreted through the urethra. The act of urine discharge is called **micturition.**

The kidneys have the following protection and coverings: fibrous capsule, perirenal fat, renal fascia, and pararenal fat.

B.

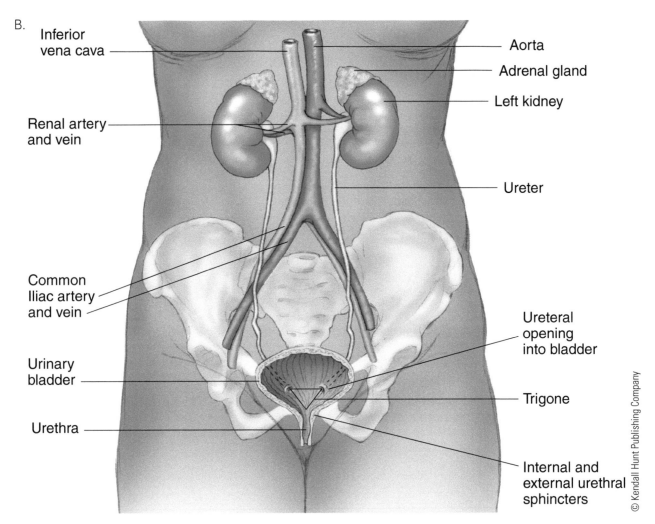

Inferior vena cava

Aorta

Adrenal gland

Left kidney

Renal artery and vein

Ureter

Common Iliac artery and vein

Ureteral opening into bladder

Urinary bladder

Trigone

Urethra

Internal and external urethral sphincters

FIGURE 21-1 Organs of the Urinary System Anterior View

C. **FUNCTIONS:** The renal system performs multiple functions, including but not limited to the following:
1. Regulation of blood volume
2. Regulation of blood ions
3. Regulation of blood pH (along with lungs)
4. Regulation of blood pressure via the production of renin (powerful vasoconstrictor)
5. Production of hormones: erythropoietin in red blood cell synthesis
6. Elimination of wastes from the body

II. Gross Anatomy of the Urinary System

A.

TABLE 21-1 Gross Anatomy: Kidney Structures

MAJOR STRUCTURES	FEATURES AND FUNCTIONS
KIDNEY COVERINGS	Protect and secure the kidneys to the posterior body wall.
■ RENAL CAPSULE	Tough fibrous capsule, outer covering of the kidney.
■ PERIRENAL FAT	Fat covering on the fibrous capsule.
■ RENAL FASCIA	Loose connective tissue outside of the perirenal fat and surrounds both the kidney and the supra-renal glands above it.
■ PARARENAL FAT	Located outside of the renal fascia. And made up of large amount of fat.
HILUM	The indent on the medial border of the kidney, and is continuous with the larger cavity **(renal sinus).** The renal pelvis, renal artery and vein, autonomic nerves, lymph nodes, and fatty tissue all can be found in the hilum.
RENAL CORTEX	Outer part. Lies beneath the capsule, overlies the bases of the pyramids and then dips downwards into the medulla and between the pyramids as **renal columns.**
RENAL MEDULLA	Inner segment, striated in appearance. The renal pyramids, collecting ducts, loops of Henle are located here.
RENAL PYRAMID	Approximately 12–18 in number. The base originates in the cortex and the apex **(renal papilla)** projects medially.
RENAL COLUMN	Are projections of the cortex into the spaces between the pyramids.
RENAL LOBULE	Consists of the renal pyramid plus the cortex area just above it.
MINOR CALYCES	Receive drainage from the collecting ducts and drain out via the renal papilla. Minors then drain into major calyces.
MAJOR CALYCES	3–5 minor calyces drain into a larger major calyx. Typically there are 3–4 major calyces per kidney.
RENAL PAPILLA	The apex of the renal pyramid and the collective opening of the collecting ducts of urine. Drains into the **minor calyces.**
RENAL PELVIS	This is the expanded upper end of the ureter within the renal sinus and hilum. The pelvis receives drainage from the major calyces.

B.

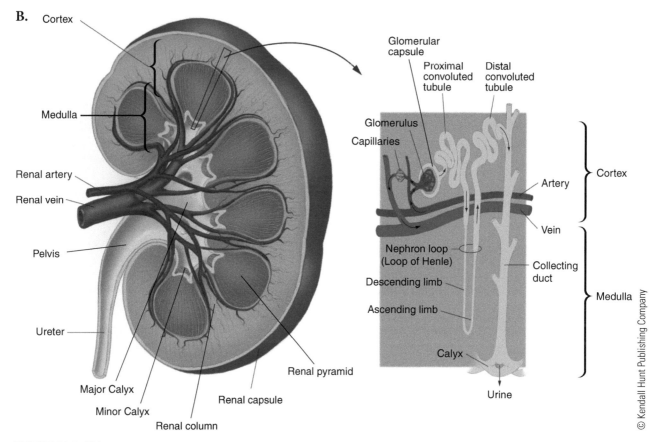

FIGURE 21-2 Kidney

C.

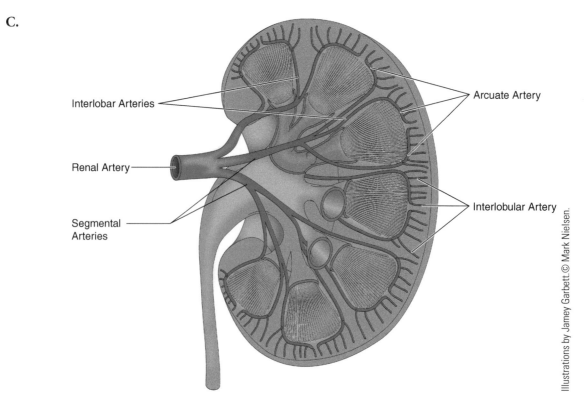

FIGURE 21-3 Arteries of the Kidney

D. Lab Activity 21-1: Identify the Structures on the Kidney and Kub Models

See the Photo Atlas

LIST OF TERMINOLOGY

- **renal vein**
- **renal artery**
- **ureter**
- **hilum**
- **cortex**
- **medulla**
- **renal pyramids**
- **renal papilla**
- **calyx (major, minor)**
- **renal papilla**
- **renal pelvis**
- **arteries:**
  - **renal, segmental, lobar, interlobar, arcuate, interlobular**
- **veins:**
  - **interlobular, arcuate, interlobar**
- **A. Identify the urethra from the male reproductive organ**

A. Lab Activity 21-2: Sheep Kidney Dissection.

IDENTIFY THESE STRUCTURES ON THE PIG/SHEEP KIDNEY

See the Photo Atlas

SHEEP KIDNEY DISSECTION INSTRUCTIONS

1. Place the preserved kidney and the dissecting instruments on a dissecting tray.

2. Identify the following external gross structures: renal capsule, hilum, renal artery, renal vein, and ureter.

3. Make a longitudinal and lengthwise (frontal section) cut on the kidney, then identify the following structures:

LIST OF TERMINOLOGY:

- **Renal vein**
- **Renal artery**
- **ureter**
- **hilum**
- **cortex**
- **medulla**
- **renal pyramids**
- **renal papilla**
- **calyx (major, minor)**
- **renal pelvis**
- **arteries (IF your kidney is injected with latex):**
  - **renal, segmental, lobar, interlobar, arcuate, interlobular**
- **veins: (IF your kidney is injected with latex):**
  - **interlobular, arcuate, interlobar, renal**

III. The Nephron

A.

TABLE 21-2 Parts of the Nephron

MAJOR NEPHRON SEGMENTS	FEATURES	FUNCTIONS
GLOMERULUS CAPILLARIES	Formed by the incoming larger **afferent arteriole** and is made up of tangled capillaries within the Bowman capsule. Blood leaves the capillary via smaller **efferent arteriole.**	Hydrostatic blood pressure drives plasma and waste materials through the filtration membrane.
GLOMERULUS (BOWMAN) CAPSULE	The proximal end of the nephron, shaped like a bowl (covered). The glomerulus capillary is located within it. This capsule ("bowl") has 2 layers: outer parietal and inner visceral. The visceral layer is sticky to the glomerulus below and the 2 forms the respiratory membrane.	Houses the glomerulus and receives the filtrate.
FILTRATION MEMBRANE	Formed by **3 structures**: **1.** the visceral layer (it's podocytic cell) of the Bowman capsule, **2.** the endothelium of the glomerulus capillary, and **3.** their basement membranes fused together in between them.	Filtration of plasma content takes place here. The filtrate flows into PCT.
RENAL CORPUSCLE	The complex of glomerulus plus the glomerulus (Bowman) capsule. Located in the cortex of the kidney.	
PROXIMAL CONVOLUTED TUBULE	The proximal segment of the nephron tube, and closer to the glomerulus capsule.	**Reabsorption** of water (passive), amino acids and glucose (active) from the lumen into surrounding capillaries (peritubular capillaries). **Secretion** of H+, K+, drugs (active) from peritubular capillaries into the nephron lumen.
DESCENDING LOOP	Descending limb of the loop of Henle.	Highly permeable to water only. Reabsorption of water (passive) from the lumen into surrounding capillaries (vasa recta).
ASCENDING LOOP	Ascending limb of loop of Henle.	Permeable to salt only. Reabsorption of salt (active) from the lumen into surrounding capillaries (vasa recta).
DISTAL CONVOLUTED TUBULE	Distal segment of the nephron is continuous with collecting tubule below.	**Reabsorption** of water (passive), amino acids and glucose (active) from the lumen into surrounding capillaries (peritubular capillaries). **Secretion** of H+, K+, drugs (active) from peritubular capillaries into the nephron lumen. The hormones ADH and aldosterone work here and in the collecting duct.

MAJOR NEPHRON SEGMENTS	FEATURES	FUNCTIONS
COLLECTING DUCT	Multiple nephrons drain their products into this. After further reabsorption, urine is the final product leaving into minor calyx.	Reabsorption of water, urea (passive), and NaCl (active). The hormones ADH and aldosterone act here.
PAPILLA	Opening of the collecting ducts into the minor calyx. It is also at the apex of the pyramid.	Draining from collecting duct into minor calyx.

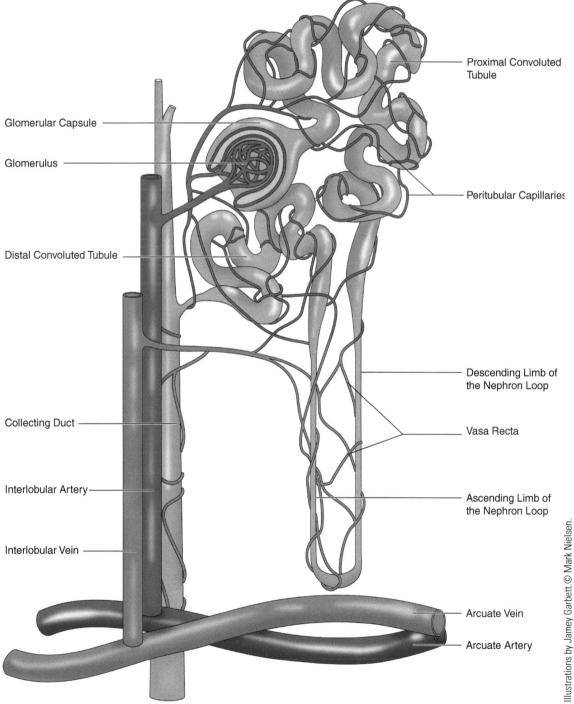

Glomerular Capsule

Glomerulus

Distal Convoluted Tubule

Collecting Duct

Interlobular Artery

Interlobular Vein

Proximal Convoluted Tubule

Peritubular Capillaries

Descending Limb of the Nephron Loop

Vasa Recta

Ascending Limb of the Nephron Loop

Arcuate Vein

Arcuate Artery

Illustrations by Jamey Garbett. © Mark Nielsen.

FIGURE 21-4 Nephron

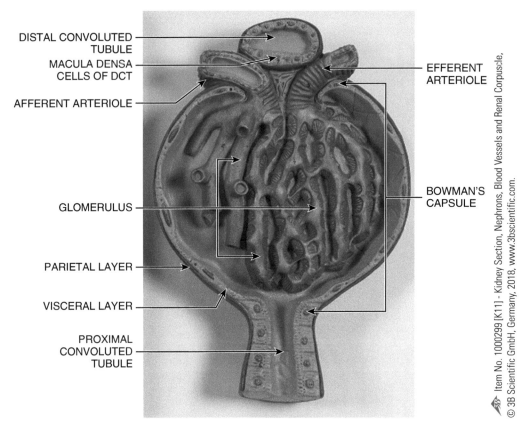

DISTAL CONVOLUTED TUBULE

MACULA DENSA CELLS OF DCT

AFFERENT ARTERIOLE

EFFERENT ARTERIOLE

BOWMAN'S CAPSULE

GLOMERULUS

PARIETAL LAYER

VISCERAL LAYER

PROXIMAL CONVOLUTED TUBULE

Item No. 1000299 [K11] - Kidney Section, Nephrons, Blood Vessels and Renal Corpuscle, © 3B Scientific GmbH, Germany, 2018, www.3bscientific.com.

FIGURE 21-5 Renal Corpuscle

B. Blood Flow at the Level of Nephron:

TABLE 21-3 Blood Flow Through the Nephron

BLOOD VESSELS	FEATURES
AFFERENT ARTERIOLE	This is the incoming larger arteriole into the glomerulus. Supply oxygenated blood to the glomerulus.
GLOMERULUS	Tangled capillary bed formed by the afferent arteriole. Is located within Bowman capsule. These are fenestrated capillaries.
EFFERENT ARTERIOLE	Outgoing smaller arterioles carry blood from the capillary bed. It would become **1. peritubular capillaries** around the PCT and DCT or **2. vasa recta capillaries** around the loop of Henle in the medulla.
PERITUBULAR CAPILLARIES	A continuation of the efferent arteriole. Surrounds cortical nephrons at the PCT and DCT.
VASA RECTA	A continuation of the efferent arteriole. It surrounds the loops of Henle of juxtamedullary nephrons.
INTERLOBULAR VEINS	Exit vessel, drain the capillaries around the nephron, and would eventually become larger renal vein.

KIDNEY BLOOD FLOW THROUGH THE NEPHRON:

Renal Artery → Segmental a. → Interlobar a. → Arcade (cortico-radiate) a. → Interlobular a. → Afferent a. → Efferent a. → Peritubular capillaries (or Vasa Recta) Interlobular v. → Arcade (cortico-radiate) v. → Interlobar a. → Segmental a. → Renal v.

C. **Lab Activity 21-3: Identify the Structures on the Kidney Nephron**

See the Photo Atlas

A. View A Microscope Slide Of Kidney

LIST OF TERMINOLOGY: Identify These Structures:

Renal lobule
Renal corpuscle
Loop of Henle (descending, ascending)
Collecting duct
Peritubular capillaries
Renal papilla
Afferent arteriole (with juxtaglomerular (JG) cells)
Efferent arteriole
Bowman capsule (with parietal and visceral layers)
Glomerulus
■ Proximal convoluted tubule (PCT)
■ Distal convoluted tubule (DCT) with densa macula cells

IV. Processes in Urine Formation

A.

TABLE 21-4 Urine Formation

PROCESS INVOLVED	DEFINITION/FEATURES	LOCATION(S)
FILTRATION	The movement of materials from fenestrated blood capillaries (of glomerulus) across the filtration membrane into the Bowman capsule. The product is called filtrate.	Glomerulus of the Bowman capsule only
REABSORPTION	Solutes in the filtrate are reabsorbed from the lumen across the nephron wall into blood (peritubular capillaries and vasa recta). Transport processes such as active transport, and facilitated and passive diffusion are involved.	All segments of the nephron
SECRETION	Solutes are secreted from blood capillaries across the nephron wall into nephron lumen (opposite reabsorption). Active transport is involved (ATP).	PCT and mostly in DCT
EXCRETION/ ELIMINATION	Movement of formed urine with waste products from the kidney to the exterior.	Ureters, bladder, and urethra

B.

I)

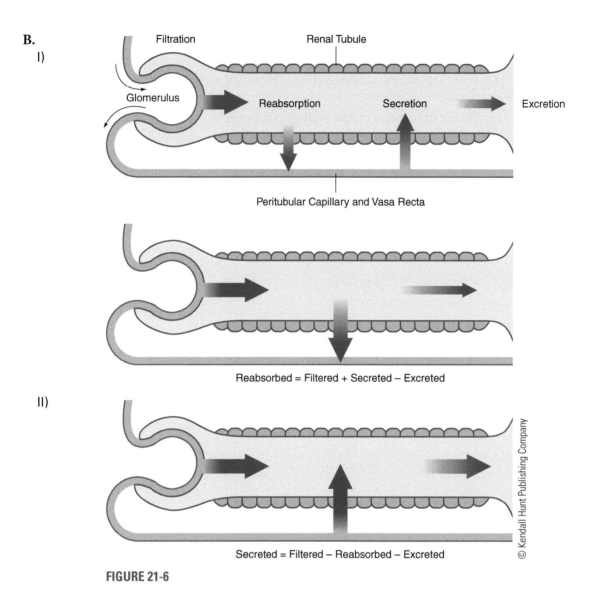

II)

FIGURE 21-6

V. Urine Flow: From Ureter to the Outside

A. URETER: Paired muscular tubes extend from the kidney pelvis and enter the posterior aspect of the cystic bladder. The junction of the ureter and bladder is called the **ureterovesical junction (UVJ).** Some patients with recurrent bladder infections may have reflux of urine from bladder back into the ureter because of abnormal UVJ.

B.

TABLE 21-5 Bladder Structures

STRUCTURES	FEATURES
DETRUSOR MUSCLES	Set of smooth muscles that form the bladder wall. During micturition (urination), which is under autonomic stimulation, the detrusor contracts to expel urine through the sphincters (internal and external) and into the urethra.
RUGAE	Multiple mucosa folds allow for expansion of the bladder during stretch.
TRIGONE	The smooth triangle-shaped area. Its base is formed by the 2 ureteral orifice/ opening (into the bladder) and the apex (or anterior angle) by the internal orifice of the urethra. The apex is toward the pubic symphysis. The base is at the fundus of the bladder.

C. **URETHRA:** The conduit (tube) that leads from the bladder to the outside. In males it is longer, and has three parts: prostatic, membranous, and spongy urethra. It functions for both urine and sperm transfer. In females it is very short in length (1.5 in. or 3.8 cm) and exits from the bladder below the clitoris.

D. **LAB ACTVITY 21-4: IDENTIFY BLADDER AND URETHRA STRUCTURES**

See the Photo Atlas

  i) KUB Stand and Male/Female Reproductive Models.

  ii) LIST OF TERMINOLGY:

   ■ **rugae**

   ■ **trigone**

   ■ **urethra**

   ■ **sphincter (internal)**

   ■ **sphincter (external) or urogenital diaphragm**

   ■ **UVJ (Ureter-Vessical junction)**

VI. Urinalysis Compared: Normal versus Abnormal

A.

TABLE 21-6 Urinalysis: Normal Versus Abnormal

SUBSTANCE	NORMAL URINE	PATHOLOGICAL FINDINGS (IF PRESENT)/CAUSES
BLOOD	None	Glomerulonephritis, renal calculi, cystitis (bladder), urethritis, or cancer.
PROTEIN	None	Glomerulonephritis, diabetic nephropathy.
GLUCOSE	None	Glomerulonephritis, diabetic nephropathy.
BLOOD UREA NITROGEN (BUN)	Trace	Higher levels: dehydration or renal failure.
KETONES	None	Diabetic nephropathy, from fatty acid metabolism in diabetic patients.
KETOACIDS	None	Diabetic nephropathy, from amino acid metabolism in diabetic patients.
PUS	None	Pyelonephritis, serious bacterial infection of the kidney.

VII. Clinical Applications in Renal Diseases

A.

TABLE 21-7 Clinical Application in Renal System

DISEASE/CONDITIONS	DEFINITION/SYMPTOMS	DIAGNOSIS/TREATMENT
GLOMERULONEPHRITIS	Inflammation of the glomerulus complex. Caused by autoimmune disease or bacteria.	Urinalysis and patient history. Treatment: antibiotic, steroids, and immune suppression.
■ ACUTE	Follows bacteria strep infection. Fever, chill, edema of the hands and feet/face, hematuria, and albuminuria.	Same as above.
■ CHRONIC	Often caused by autoimmune disease. Remission and exacerbation of symptoms. Uremia is obvious. May lead to renal failure.	Same as above.
PYELONEPHRITIS	Blood-borne infection and pus formation of the kidney. Leading to high fever, chills, pyuria (pus in the urine), hematuria, and renal failure.	Urinalysis. Treatment: IV fluids and antibiotics.
RENAL FAILURE		
■ ACUTE	Often resulting from incompatible blood transfusion, other toxins or drug toxicity, and severe shock from sudden blood loss. Symptoms of oliguria and anuria.	Patient history, urinalysis, blood. Treatment: drugs, fluids, antibiotics, and possible dialysis.
■ CHRONIC	Commonly from hypertension, diabetic nephropathy, and chronic glomerulonephritis. Anuria and edema.	Patient history, urinalysis, blood. Treatment: dialysis and transplant.
URINARY CALCULI (STONES)	Most commonly due to excess calcium deposition in kidneys, flank pain that radiates to groin.	Urinalysis, X-ray, IV pyelogram. Treatment: lithotripsy or surgery.
HYDRONEPHROSIS	Dilated ureter (water in the ureter) secondary to renal obstruction. Pain, hematuria.	Urinalysis, IV pyelogram. Treatment: surgery.
POLYCYSTIC KIDNEY	Genetic. Symptoms include hypertension, renal failure, and uremia.	Urinalysis, IV pyelogram. Treatment: surgery (kidney transplant).
CARCINOMA (EXAMPLE BLADDER)	Unknown causes, smoking history. Hematuria, pelvic pain, and frequent urination.	Cystoscopy. Surgery.

VIII. Post-Lab Activity: Renal (Label these Structures)

A.

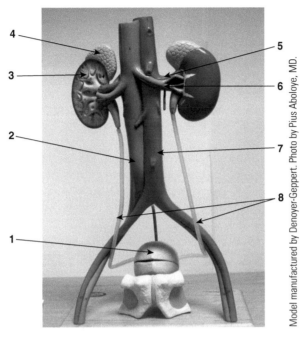

Model manufactured by Denoyer-Geppert. Photo by Pius Aboloye, MD.

FIGURE 21-7 Renal System Anatomy (Anterior View)

B.

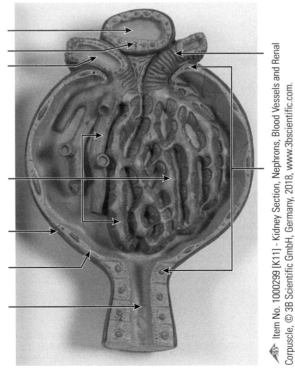

Item No. 1000299 [K11] - Kidney Section, Nephrons, Blood Vessels and Renal Corpuscle, © 3B Scientific GmbH, Germany, 2018, www.3bscientific.com.

FIGURE 21-8 Renal Corpuscle

C.

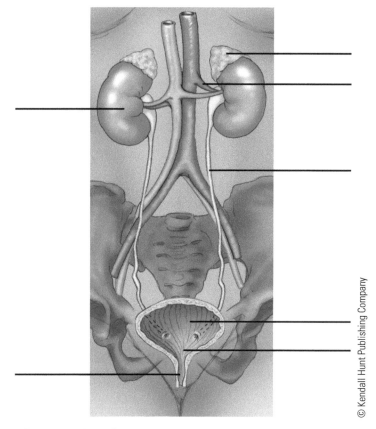

FIGURE 21-9 Renal System Anatomy Anterior

D.

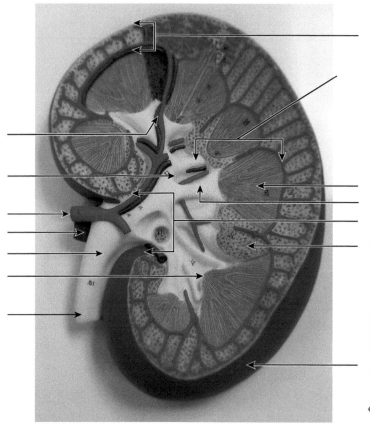

FIGURE 21-10 Kidney and Nephron Anatomy

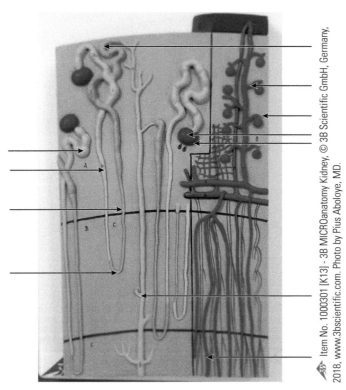

Item No. 1000301 [K13] - 3B MICROanatomy Kidney, © 3B Scientific GmbH, Germany, 2018, www.3bscientific.com. Photo by Pius Aboloye, MD.

FIGURE 21-11 Kidney Lobule and Nephron Anatomy

A. Complete the following:

  1. All of the following are functions of the renal system except

    A. elimination of organic wastes

    B. regulation of red blood synthesis

    C. regulation of blood volume and pH

    D. production of ADH

  2. The triangle-shaped area within the urinary bladder is called

    A. urethral opening

    B. trigone

    C. mucosa fold

    D. detrusor muscle

  3. The glomerulus plus the Bowman capsule is called

    A. renal corpuscle

    B. renal tubule

    C. renal capsule

    D. renal pelvis

  4. The urinary system consists of all of the following except

    A. ureter

    B. urethra

    C. kidney

    D. gallbladder

5. The cone-like structure in the renal medulla plus the cortex above it is referred to as
   A. renal column
   B. renal lobule
   C. renal pelvis
   D. renal pyramid

6. Identify this hormone that is produced by the kidneys
   A. ADH
   B. aldosterone
   C. thymosin
   D. erythropoietin

7. List the sequence of urine flow from the collecting duct to the outside.

8. List the regions of the nephron.

9. List the correct sequence of blood flow (arterial and venous) through the kidney.

10. Distinguish between cortico-nephrons and juxtamedullary-type nephrons.

11. Make a list of the structures that can be found in the renal hilum.

Male Reproductive System

Upon completion of this exercise, you should be able to:

A. Describe the major functions of the reproductive system.
B. Identify the gross and microscopic features of the male and female organs.
C. Identify the accessory structures and functions of both male and female organs.
D. List the parts of the male urethra.
E. List the main blood vessels of the reproductive system.
F. Describe the ductal system in both male and female organs.
G. List the clinical applications.

NEEDED MATERIALS

1. Human torso: pelvis.
2. Models: male and female models.
3. Male reproductive organ (for urethra identification).
4. Microscope slides: testis, sperm smear, ovary, and uterus.

Introduction

I. OVERVIEW

A. The reproductive system includes the primary organs, the duct system, and other accessory glands:
   i) **Primary organs** include paired testis (male) and paired ovaries (female) because they produce the gametes and hormones.
   ii) **Ductal system** includes the tubes that conduct or transfer the gametes or semen.
   iii) **Accessory glands and organs** produce secretions that aid in the transfer of gametes, and external genitalia.

B

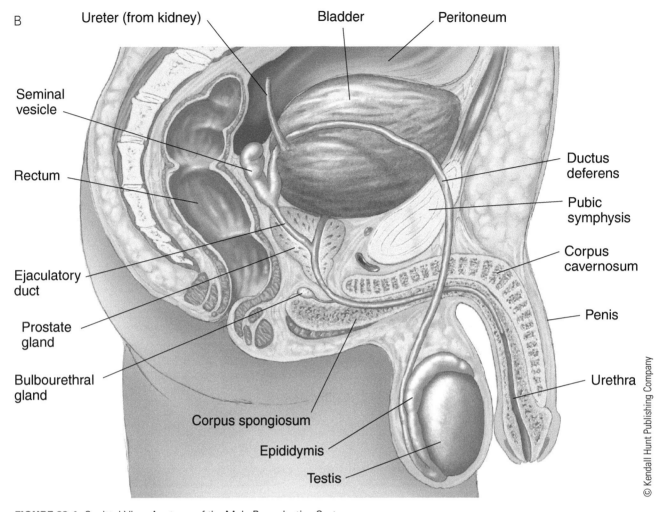

Ureter (from kidney)

Bladder

Peritoneum

Seminal vesicle

Rectum

Ejaculatory duct

Prostate gland

Bulbourethral gland

Corpus spongiosum

Epididymis

Testis

Ductus deferens

Pubic symphysis

Corpus cavernosum

Penis

Urethra

FIGURE 22-1 Sagittal View Anatomy of the Male Reproductive System

C. **FUNCTIONS:** The reproductive system performs multiple functions including the following:
1. Gamete production (ova and spermatozoa)
2. Fertilization
3. Production of reproductive hormones (testosterone, estrogen, and progesterone)
4. Development and nourishment of the fetus (in females)

II. Gross Anatomy of the Male Reproductive System

A.

TABLE 22-1 **External Male Reproductive Organ System**

STRUCTURE	FEATURES AND FUNCTIONS
PENIS	The organ of copulation in the male. Functions in the introduction of sperms into the female reproductive tract. Consist of 3 erectile tissues.
■ CORPUS CARVONOSA (2)	2 cylindrical erectile penile tissues located on the dorsal aspect.
■ CORPUS SPONGIOSUM (1)	1 cylindrical erectile penile tissue located on the ventral aspect. The spongy urethra passes through this on the ventral aspect.
GLANS	The expanded distal end of the erectile tissue.
PREPUCE	The hood-like foreskin on the glans penis. **Circumcision** is the removal of the prepuce.
SPONGY URETHRA	Part of the urethra that passes through the corpus spongiosum on the ventral aspect on the penis.
TESTES	The primary organ of reproduction in the male; produces hormones and gametes.
DARTOS MUSCLE	Smooth muscle found in the subcutaneous of the scrotum, the skin when it contracts.
CREMASTER MUSCLES	Bundle of skeletal muscles found deeper in the scrotal sac and continuous in the spermatic cord. When stimulated, elevates the testes toward the body for warmth.
EPIDIDYMIS	C-shaped atop the testis. Acts as storage and maturation site for the spermatozoa. It is continuous with the vas deferens.
SPERMATIC CORD	Contents: vas deferens, testicular artery, pampiniform plexus of veins, lymphatics, autonomic nerves.

B.

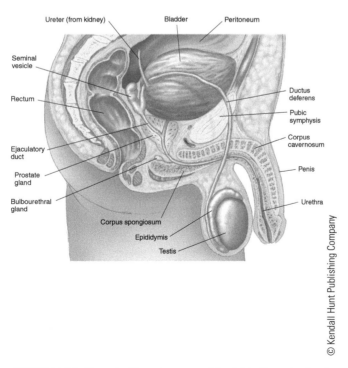

FIGURE 22-2 Posterior View Anatomy of the Male Reproductive System

C. Lab Activity 22-1: Identify the structures on the male model and torso

See the Photo Atlas

LIST OF TERMINOLOGY: External Features (Male):

- scrotum
- tunica albuginea
- tunica vaginalis
- Dartos muscle
- cremaster muscle
- testes
- spermatic cord and contents
- testicular a. & v.
- penis
- glans penis
- prepuce
- corpora cavernosa
- corpus spongiosum
- spongy urethra
- gonadal arteries and veins

D. **BLOOD SUPPLY:**

TESTIS: Testicular arteries (from abdominal aorta) to the testes and testicular veins (drains into the inferior vena cava.

PENIS: Dorsal arteries from the internal pudendal artery (internal iliac artery branch) and the pampiniform veins drain into internal pudendal veins (internal iliac veins).

E. **NERVE SUPPLY**

PENIS: From pudendal nerve (S2–S5 plexus) and autonomics from hypogastric and pelvic plexus.

F. **ERECTION:** It is a parasympathetic control resulting from the contraction of erectile tissues (bulbospongiosus and ischiocavernosus muscles). This compresses and traps the pampiniform veins within the penis. And concurrent increase in blood pressure and dilation of arteries increases blood flow into the spaces of the erectile tissue.

G. **EJACULATION:** It is a sympathetic control. Reflex wave of contraction of smooth muscles of the vas deferens, with contraction of seminal and prostate glands, results in emission of semen.

III. Testis

A.

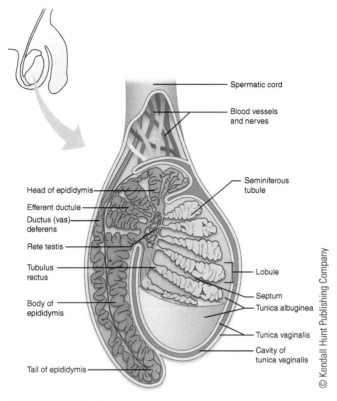

Spermatic cord

Blood vessels and nerves

Head of epididymis

Efferent ductule

Ductus (vas) deferens

Rete testis

Tubulus rectus

Body of epididymis

Tail of epididymis

Seminiferous tubule

Lobule

Septum

Tunica albuginea

Tunica vaginalis

Cavity of tunica vaginalis

© Kendall Hunt Publishing Company

FIGURE 22-3 Testis

B. Lab Activity 22-2: Describe spermatogenesis, ductal system, and sperm flow

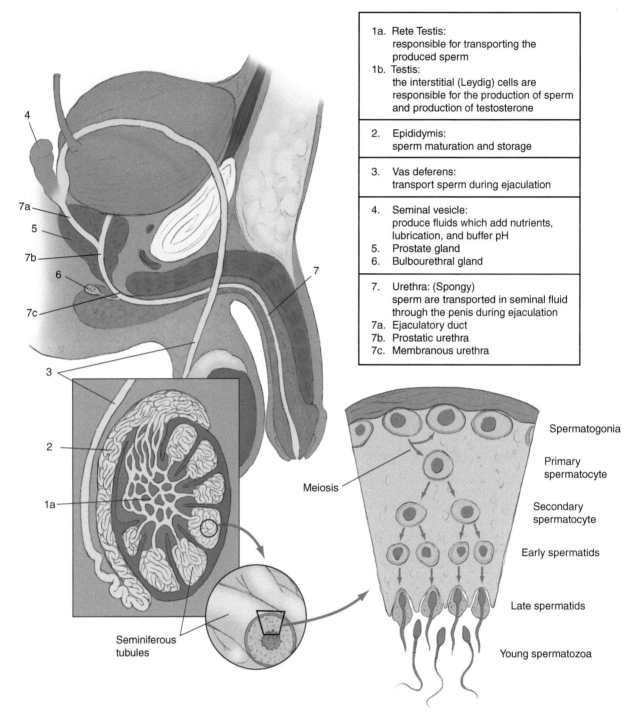

1a. Rete Testis:
responsible for transporting the
produced sperm
1b. Testis:
the interstitial (Leydig) cells are
responsible for the production of sperm
and production of testosterone

2. Epididymis:
sperm maturation and storage

3. Vas deferens:
transport sperm during ejaculation

4. Seminal vesicle:
produce fluids which add nutrients,
lubrication, and buffer pH
5. Prostate gland
6. Bulbourethral gland

7. Urethra: (Spongy)
sperm are transported in seminal fluid
through the penis during ejaculation
7a. Ejaculatory duct
7b. Prostatic urethra
7c. Membranous urethra

Spermatogonia

Primary
spermatocyte

Meiosis

Secondary
spermatocyte

Early spermatids

Late spermatids

Young spermatozoa

Seminiferous
tubules

FIGURE 22-4 Testis and Sperm Flow

- Ductal system and sperm flow:

  Seminiferous tubule Tubulus rectus (straight) Rete testes Efferent ductules Epididymis Vas deference Ejaculatory duct Urethra {Prostate, membranous, Spongy}

C. **Identify sperm structure:**

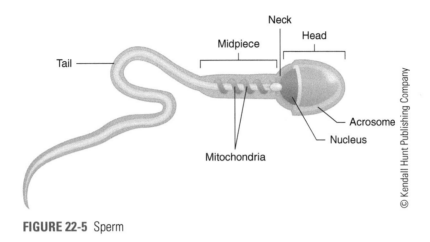

FIGURE 22-5 Sperm

- View a microscope slide of testes and sperm smear

D. **LAB ACTVITY 22-3: See the Photo Atlas**

LIST OF TERMINOLOGY:

DUCTAL SYSTEM AND SPERM FLOW	GLANDS
Seminiferous tubules (relate to lecture)	Prostate gland ■ seminal vesicles ■ bulbourethral (Cowper) glands
Rete testis	Sperm
Tubulus rectus	■ Head (with acrosome and nucleus) ■ Mid-piece ■ Tail
Efferent ducts (vasa efferentia)	
Epididymis	
Vas (ductus) deferens	
Ampulla of vas deferens	
Common ejaculatory duct	
Urethra: (prostatic, membranous, and spongy)	
External urethral orifice	

IV. Lab Activity 22-4: Identify Structure of the Penis

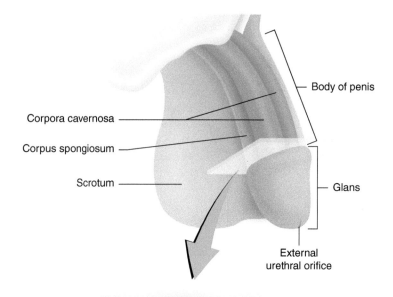

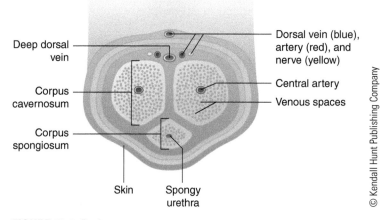

FIGURE 22-6 Penis

V. Accessory Glands

A.

TABLE 22-2 Accessory Glands (Males)

STRUCTURE	FEATURES AND FUNCTIONS
SEMINAL VESICLES	A bilobed gland. Located on the posterior aspect of the bladder. Its duct joins with the duct of the vas deference and forms **the ejaculatory duct** as it travels through the prostate gland. **Secretion consists of alkaline pH (high pH), with fructose, fibrinogen, and coagulase enzymes.** **Contributes 60% to the semen fluid in each ejaculate.**
PROSTATE	Cone-shaped glandular tissue with smooth muscles. Its base surrounds the neck of the bladder and the urethra. Its ducts open into the prostate urethra. The prostate (posterior lobe) is anterior to the rectum. Digital rectal exam is used to evaluate the prostate for cancer or enlargement. **Secretion consists of high pH, milky secretion, clotting factors, and fibrinolysin.** **Contributes 40% to the semen fluid in each ejaculate.**
BULBOURETHRA (COWPER'S GLAND)	2 small glands located along the external sphincter (urogenital diaphragm), and their ducts open into the membranous urethra. **Secretion: mucous, released prior to ejaculation and helps neutralize acid urine in the male urethra and acidity in the vagina.** **Contributes 0%–5% to the semen fluid in each ejaculate.**
SEMEN (SEMINAL FLUID)	Approximately 2–5 ml per ejaculate. Consist of millions of spermatozoa plus semen fluid.

B.

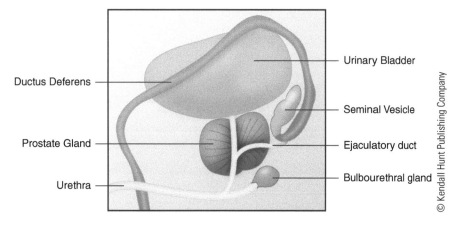

FIGURE 22-7 Accessory Glands

VI. Clinical Applications: Diseases of the Male Reproductive Tract

A.

TABLE 22-3 Clinical Application in Male System

DISEASE/CONDITION	DEFINITION/SYMPTOMS	DIAGNOSIS/TREATMENT
ORCHITIS	Inflammation of the testes often secondary to mumps (viral) infection of the parotid salivary glands. Complications include infertility.	Antibiotics.
CRYPTORCHIDISM	Failure to descend into the scrotal sac by one of or both testes. Common in premature births. May lead to increased risk for infertility and testicular cancer.	Surgery.
VASECTOMY	Surgical removal of part of the vas deferens (close to the epididymis) to prevent sperm transfer. A voluntarily means of sterilization.	None.
ERECTILE DYSFUNCTION	Inability to start or maintain an erection, most commonly due to other medical conditions: vascular diseases (diabetes, hypertension, smoking history). May be psychological.	Treatment: drugs.
TESTICULAR CANCER	Testicular mass, risk factors: family history, undescended testis.	Sonogram and CT scan. Treatment: surgery +/- adjuvant chemotherapy.
PROSTATE CANCER	Second most common cancer in males (lung #1). Hematuria. Slow metastasis.	Abnormal digital rectal exam (DRE). Elevated PSA levels. Prescreening with levels of serum prostate antigen. Treatment: surgery.
BENIGN PROSTATE ENLARGEMENT	Non-cancerous enlargement of the prostate. This then compresses the urethra (prostatic portion), leading to urinary obstruction, recurrent infections, and inability to initiate or maintain urine stream.	Abnormal DRE. Treatment: surgery when medications fail.

VII. Post-Lab Activity: Male Reproductive System
(Label these Structures)

A.

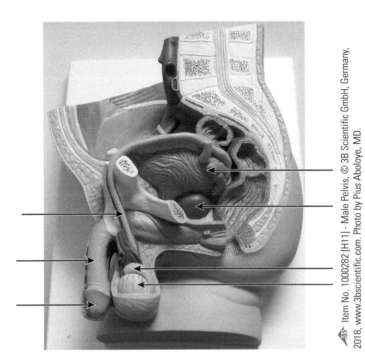

FIGURE 22-8 Male Reproductive

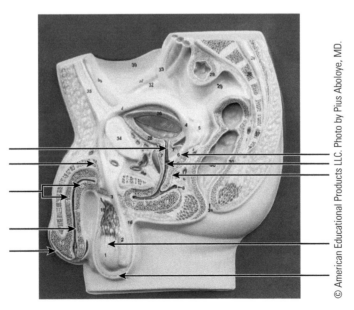

FIGURE 22-9 Male Pelvic Sagittal view

A. Answer the following questions:

1. The male urethra passes through
   A. corpus cavernosa
   B. prepuce
   C. corpus spongiosum
   D. scrotum

2. The skin fold atop the glans penis is called the
   A. corpus cavernosa
   B. prepuce
   C. corpus spongiosum
   D. scrotum

3. The spermatic cord consists of all of the following except
   A. ejaculatory duct
   B. ductus deferens
   C. blood vessels
   D. autonomic nerves

4. Interstitial (Leydig) cells of the testis produce
   A. estrogen
   B. sperm cells
   C. testosterone
   D. progesterone

5. The comma-shaped structure atop of the testes is called
   A. vas deferens
   B. seminiferous tubules
   C. epididymis
   D. rete testes

6. Sperm synthesis takes place in the:
   A. prostate
   B. seminal vesicle
   C. seminiferous tubules
   D. bulbourethral gland

7. This accessory gland produces 60% of the male ejaculate
   A. prostate gland
   B. seminal vesicle gland
   C. seminiferous tubules
   D. bulbourethral gland

8. This part of the male urethra is located within the pelvic diaphragm:
   A. prostatic urethra
   B. spongy urethra
   C. membranous urethra
   D. bulbourethral urethra

9. Describe sperm flow from seminiferous tubule and through the female reproductive tract up to fertilization.

10. Define the term phimosis.

11. List the three regions of the male urethra.

12. List the three accessory glands of the male reproductive tract and their secretions.

Female Reproductive System

Upon completion of this exercise, you should be able to:

A. Describe the major functions of the reproductive system.
B. Identify the gross and microscopic features of the male and female organs.
C. Identify the accessory structures and functions of both male and female organs.
D. List the parts of the male urethra.
E. List the main blood vessels of the reproductive system.
F. Describe the ductal system in both male and female organs.
G. List the clinical applications.

NEEDED MATERIALS

1. Human torso: pelvis.
2. Models: male and female models.
3. Male reproductive organ (for urethra identification).
4. Microscope slides: testis, sperm smear, ovary, and uterus.

Introduction

I. OVERVIEW

A. The reproductive system includes the primary organs, the duct system, and other accessory glands:
   i) **Primary organs** include paired testis (male) and paired ovaries (female) because they produce the gametes and hormones.
   ii) **Ductal system** includes the tubes that conduct or transfer the gametes or semen.
   iii) **Accessory glands and organs** produce secretions that aid in the transfer of gametes, and external genitalia.

B.

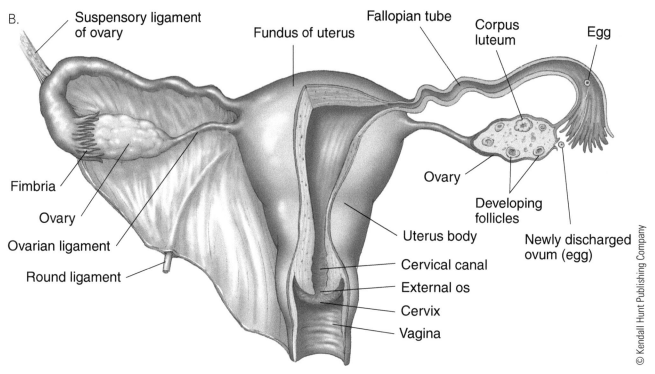

FIGURE 23-1 Anatomy of the Female Reproductive System

C. **FUNCTIONS:** The reproductive system performs multiple functions including the following:
1. Gamete production (ova and spermatozoa)
2. Fertilization
3. Production of reproductive hormones (testosterone, estrogen, and progesterone)
4. Development and nourishment of the fetus (in females)

II. Gross Anatomy of the Female Reproductive System

A.

TABLE 23-1 External Female Genitalia (Vulva)

STRUCTURE	FEATURES
PERINEUM	The diamond-shaped area between the thighs, from the mons pubis to the ischial tuberosity and posterior to the sacrum.
VULVA	Another name for external genitalia. Includes mons pubis, labia majora and minora, the clitoris, and the greater vestibular glands (mucus).
MONS PUBIS	The fatty tissue atop of the pubic symphysis, covered with hair.
LABIA MAJORA	Large folds of skin with hair, start from the mons pubis going posteriorly until the meet at midline. Is analogous to the scrotum in males.
LABIA MINORA	2 smaller skin folds with no hair. Below is the vestibule.
VESTIBULE OF THE VAGINA	This is the space between the labia minora. The apex of the vestibule has clitoris and urethra opening. Others: ducts of the greater vestibular glands and vagina.
PREPUCE	Covers the glans of the clitoris.
CLITORIS	Is analogous to the male penis. Lies superior to the urethral orifice.
URETHRA	Shorter (1.5 in. or 4 cm) compared with the male. Extends from the neck of the bladder through the urogenital diaphragm and opens to the outside just below the clitoris but anterior to the vagina.

B.

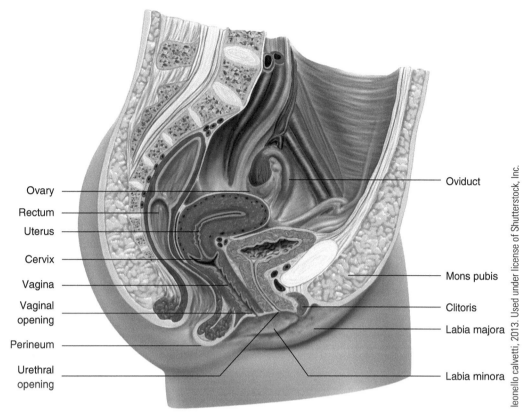

Ovary

Rectum

Uterus

Cervix

Vagina

Vaginal opening

Perineum

Urethral opening

Oviduct

Mons pubis

Clitoris

Labia majora

Labia minora

leonello calvetti, 2013. Used under license of Shutterstock, Inc.

FIGURE 23-2 Sagittal View Anatomy of the Female Reproductive System

C. Lab Activity 23-1: Identify the structures on the female model and torso

See the Photo Atlas: Female model and tissue slide

LIST OF TERMINOLOGY: External Features (Female):

- mons pubis
- perineum
- prepuce of clitoris
- clitoris
- vulva
- labia majora
- labia minora
- vagina
- greater vestibular glands
- ovarian arteries and veins

D. BLOOD SUPPLY:

OVARY: Ovarian arteries (from abdominal aorta) and ovarian veins drain into the inferior vena cava.

UTERUS: Uterine arteries (from the internal iliac artery) and the pampiniform veins drain into internal pudendal veins (internal iliac veins).

E. NERVE SUPPLY:

OVARY: From hypogastric ovarian plexus of nerves.

UTERUS: Hypogastric plexus of nerves.

VAGINA: Hypogastric plexus of nerves.

III. Ovary

A.

Ovary

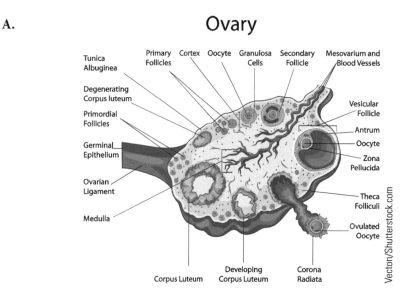

FIGURE 23-3A Ovary C/S

B. OOOGENESIS, DUCTAL SYSTEM, AND SPERM FLOW

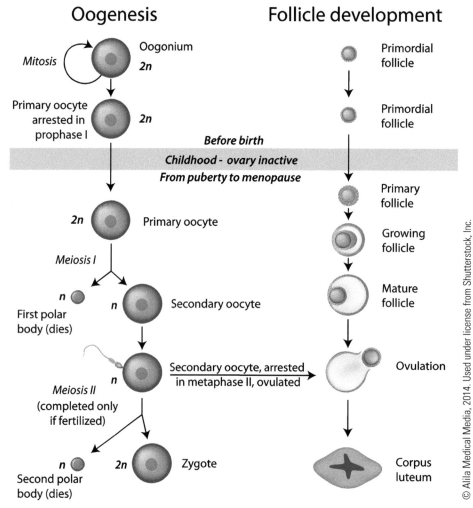

FIGURE 23-3B Oogenesis

■ Ductal system and sperm flow in the female reproductive tract:

Vagina cervix uterine cavity uterine tubes Distal 1/3 (Ampula) for Fertilization

C. OVARY STRUCTURE:

■ View a microscope slide of the ovary

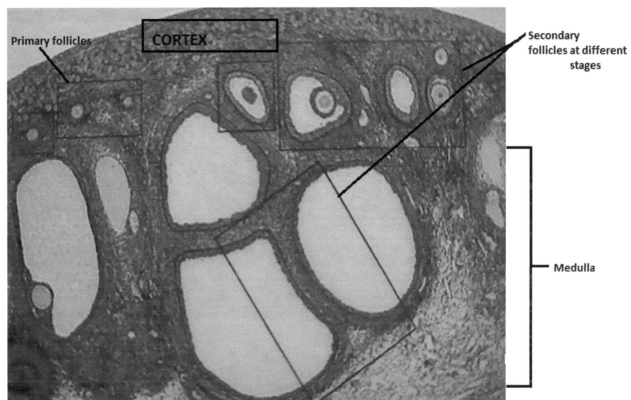

The Ovary (c/s) at different follicular growth phases

FIGURE 23-4

Photo by Pius Aboloye, MD.

LIST OF TERMINOLOGY: Female ductal system and sperm flow:

■ vagina
■ cervix (external os)
■ cervical canal
■ uterus
■ uterine (fallopian) tubes
■ infundibulum
■ isthmus
■ fimbriae

IV. Ligaments and Membranes

A.

TABLE 23-2 Parts of the Female Uterus and Tubes

STRUCTURE	FEATURES
FUNDUS	Anterior-superior aspect of the uterus.
BODY	Lies just posterior to the bladder. Its wall consists of 3 layers.
■ PERIMETRIUM	Outermost layer; is continuous with mesometrium (broad ligament).
■ MYOMETRIUM	Middle muscular layer of smooth muscles.
■ ENDOMETRIUM:	Innermost layer with the lumen above it. Consists of 2 layers.
■ BASAL LAYER	This layer is above the muscle (myometrium) layer.
■ FUNCTIONAL LAYER	The superficial layer of the endometrium. Responds to changes in ovarian hormones (estrogen and progesterone) as in increased or decreased growth of the layer. The functional layer is shed as menstruation (decreased estrogen) bleed.
CERVIX	Narrowed segment of the uterus from the body. It protrudes inferiorly into the vagina. Has gland that produces mucus to facilitate transfer of sperms toward the uterine cavity.
■ EXTERNAL OS	The opening of the uterus into vagina. Always closed and plugged with thick mucus except during ovulation when the mucus is thin and it slightly opens to facilitate sperm entry.
■ CERVICAL CANAL	The bridging short hallway from the uterine cavity neck or isthmus (internal os) toward the vagina below.
■ INTERNAL OS	The isthmus of uterine cavity toward the cervical canal below.
FALLOPIAN TUBES	Also known as uterine tubes or salpinx transports the ova from ovary to the uterine cavity.
FIMBRAE	These are finger-like projections of the distal fallopian tubes and in close proximity of the ovaries. Received ovulated ova from the ovary and by peristalsis and ciliary action, moves the ova into the Distal one-third of the tube where fertilization occurs.

Female Reproductive Tract
(Posterior view)

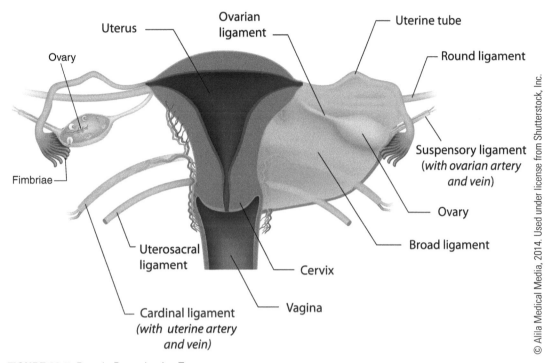

Uterus — Ovarian ligament — Uterine tube

Ovary — Round ligament

Fimbriae — Suspensory ligament (*with ovarian artery and vein*)

Ovary

Uterosacral ligament — Broad ligament

Cervix

Cardinal ligament (*with uterine artery and vein*) — Vagina

© Alila Medical Media, 2014. Used under license from Shutterstock, Inc.

FIGURE 23-5 Female Reproductive Tract

Ligaments and membranes: Identify:

■ suspensory ligament of ovary

■ ovarian ligament

■ broad ligament

■ round ligament

V. Uterus

A.

TABLE 23-3 Ligaments of the Female Reproductive System

STRUCTURE	FEATURES
BROAD LIGAMENTS (MESOMETRIUM)	Right and left sides. Each is a double layer of peritoneum fold extending from the lateral wall of uterus to the lateral and inferior pelvic walls. Contains 1. round ligaments of the ovary and uterus, 2. uterine tube, and 3. uterine and ovarian vessels and nerves.
ROUND LIGAMENTS OF THE UTERUS	Extend from the superior-lateral angle of the uterus through the inguinal canal and anchored to the labia majora. Function to keep the uterus anteverted and anterio-flexed.
OVARIAN LIGAMENTS	Rounded, cord-like thickened part of the Broad ligament, attaches the ovaries to the uterine wall. Aka utero-ovarian ligament.

B.

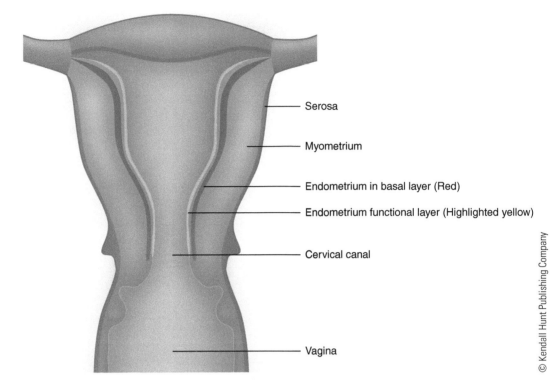

Serosa

Myometrium

Endometrium in basal layer (Red)

Endometrium functional layer (Highlighted yellow)

Cervical canal

Vagina

FIGURE 23-6 Uterine Wall

C. Lab Activity 23-4: Locate and identify these structures on the model/photos

LIST OF TERMINOLOGY: Identify Uterine Wall

- endometrium
- myometrium
- perimetrium
- menstrual cycle (ovulation)
- uterine and ovarian arteries

VI. Female Menstrual Cycle

A.

FEMALE REPRODUCTIVE CYCLES: SUMMARY OF EVENTS

	PRE-OVULATION	BIG O OVULATION DAY 14	**POST OVULATION**

**O
OVARIAN
CYCLE**
	FOLLICULAR STAGE
	❖ DAYS: 1–14
	❖ EVENT: FOLLICULAR GROWTH TO GRAFFIAN FOLLICLE (GF)
	  ○ Primary to Secondary follicle/oocyte
	❖ INITIALLY: LOW ESTROGEN
	❖ LATER: ↑ESTROGEN (from GF) inhibits FSH/LH ——→ ↑ FSH & LH
	LH surge @ DAY 12
		BIG O OVULATION DAY 14
		
		↑LH
			LUTEAL PHASE
			❖ DAYS: 14–28
			❖ EVENT: CORPUS LUTEUM ACTION
			  ○ ↑**PG** vs ESTROGEN

U UTERINE CYCLE	**MENSTRUAL PHASE** ❖ DAYS: 1–5 ❖ EVENT: SHEDDING ENDOMETRIUM **PRE-OVULATORY/ PROLIFERATIVE PHASE** ❖ DAYS: 6–14 ❖ EVENT: REBUILDING ENDOMETRIUM	**BIG O** OVULATION DAY 14	**POST-OVULATORY/ SECRETORY PHASE** ❖ DAYS: 15–28 ❖ EVENT: PREP FOR UTERINE IMPLANTATION

Source: Pius Aboloye, MD.

B.

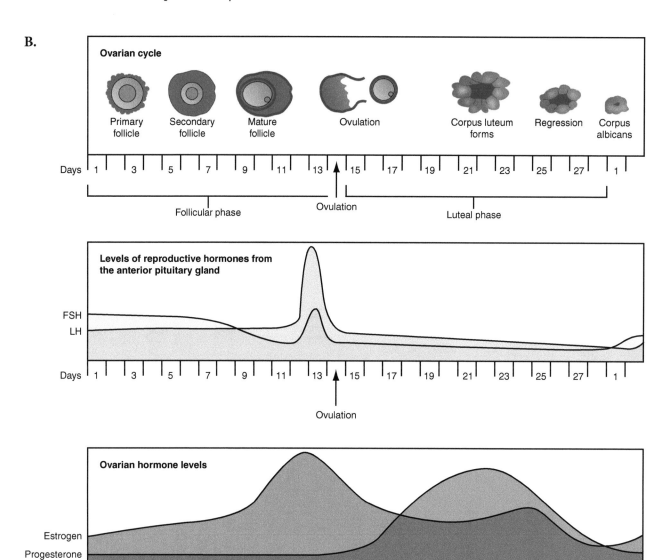

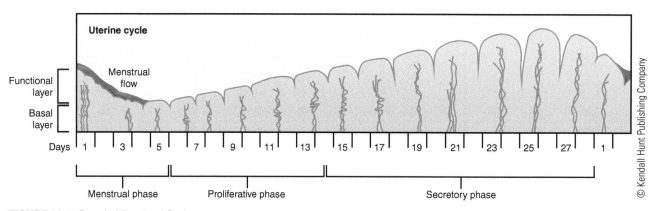

FIGURE 23-7 Female Menstrual Cycle

C.

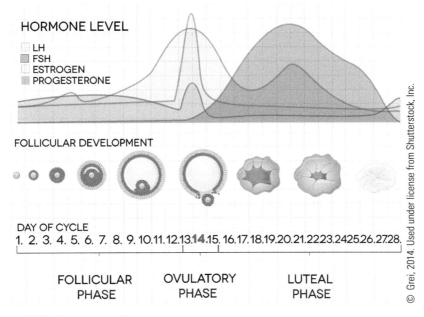

FIGURE 23-8 Female Cycle

D. Lab Activity 23-5: Locate and identify these structures on the model or photos
LIST OF TERMINOLOGY: Identify Structures of the Ovary

- cortex
- medulla
- ovarian cycle
  - primary follicle
  - secondary follicle
  - Graafian follicle
  - corpus luteum
  - corpus albicans (atretic follicle)
- oogenesis: Identify Structures of the Ovary on a diagram
  - primary oocyte
  - secondary oocyte
  - ovum

VII. The Breast

A. STRUCTURE:

The breasts are located on ribs 2 to 6. The mammary glands are modified sweat glands that produce milk. The **nipple** is a small rounded tip consisting of smooth muscle fibers that contracts upon stimulation. The **areola** is the pigmented area around the nipple.

The breast consists of 15 to 20 lobes; each is separated by **septa** (connective tissue), and further divided into **lobules and acini,** resembling a cut grapefruit. Each gland is drained by a **lactiferous duct**, which then opens into **lactiferous sinus** which opens into the nipple.

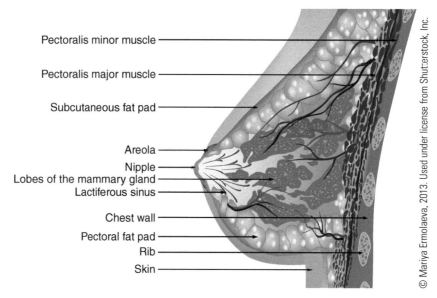

Pectoralis minor muscle

Pectoralis major muscle

Subcutaneous fat pad

Areola

Nipple

Lobes of the mammary gland

Lactiferous sinus

Chest wall

Pectoral fat pad

Rib

Skin

© Mariya Ermolaeva, 2013. Used under license from Shutterstock, Inc.

FIGURE 23-9 Breast

VIII. Clinical Applications: Diseases of Female Reproductive Tract

A.

TABLE 23-5 Clinical Application in Female System

DISEASE/CONDITION	DEFINITION/SYMPTOMS	DIAGNOSIS/TREATMENT
BARTHOLIN CYST	Cyst(s) of the major vestibular glands (mucus secreting). Located in the vestibule of the vagina. Very painful.	Pelvic exam. Excision and drainage.
EPISIOTOMY	An incision made on the vulva to control or direct tear of the perineum during active labor.	Repair is made immediately after delivery.
CERVICAL CANCER	Typically with no symptoms. History of cervical dysplasia, may present with vaginal discharge or bleeding.	Cervical examination and biopsy. Surgical excision or hysterectomy (advanced stages) +/- adjuvant chemotherapy.
ENDOMETRIOSIS	A condition where endometrium tissue is found elsewhere (ovary, fallopian tube, and outside the uterine wall or pelvic floor). Painful menstruation bleeding.	Laparoscopic ablation ("laser removal") or surgery.
FIBROIDS	Unknown cause, history of abnormal bleeding, prolonged menstruation, and pelvic pain.	Sonogram and pelvic examination. Excision or myolysis.
PELVIC INFLAMMATORY DISEASE (PID)	Secondary to genitourinary infection. Pain, fever, and chills.	Bacterial culture is positive. Treatment: antibiotics and fluids.

DISEASE/CONDITION	DEFINITION/SYMPTOMS	DIAGNOSIS/TREATMENT
OVARIAN CYST	May be single or multiple cystic growth on the ovary.	Laparoscopy. Treatment: excision and hormone therapy.
OVARIAN CANCER	Unknown causes. Low-survival rate at 5 years.	Pelvic exam. CT scan and laparoscopy with biopsy. Treatment: excision and chemo- or hormone therapy.
ECTOPIC PREGNANCY	Fertilization and implantation of the zygote in the uterine tube (most common) or pelvic cavity.	Salpingectomy and removal.
SALPINGITIS	Inflammation of the uterine tubes.	Antibiotics and/salpingectomy.
HYSTERECTOMY	Surgical removal of the uterus (partial/total) with or without **salpingectomy (fallopian tube removal)**. Often secondary to diseased uterus/cervix/ovary (cancer or severe uterine bleed).	None.
OOPHORECTOMY	Surgical removal of the ovary, bilateral or unilateral often secondary to diseased ovary (cancer or others).	None.
BREAST CANCER	Unknown causes. Palpable mass with or without lymph nodes palpable.	Mammogram and biopsy. Treatment: surgery +/- adjuvant therapy (radiation/chemo-/hormone replacement therapy [HRT]).
AMENORRHEA	No menses second low gonadotropin hormones.	Pelvic examination and hormone levels. Treatment: HRT.
DYSMENORRHEA	History of pelvic infection, endometriosis. History of painful bleeding, prolonged menstruation. Dull to severe pelvic and back pain.	Pelvic examination and laparoscopy. Treatment: Anti-inflammatory drugs, D&C, plus oral contraceptives.
MENORRHAGIA	History of excessive menstrual bleeding, commonly due to uterine fibroids, PID.	Pelvic exam. And hormone levels. Treatment: surgery (hysterectomy), endometrial ablation, antibiotic, HRT.
METRORRHAGIA	Second to hormone imbalance. Patient has history of abnormal bleeding, extremely irregular menstrual cycle.	Pelvic exam. And hormone levels. Treatment: D&C.
PREMENSTRUAL SYNDROME	Unknown causes. Collection of symptoms, including bloating, breast pain, depression, and irritability just prior to the onset of menses.	Treatment: changes in diet, increase exercise, antidepressant or hormone therapy.
MENOPAUSE	Cessation of menstruation after age 50. Hot flashes, night sweat, irritability, vaginal dryness.	High FSH and low estrogen levels. Treatment: HRT.

IX. Post-Lab Activity: Female Reproductive System: Label these Structures

A.

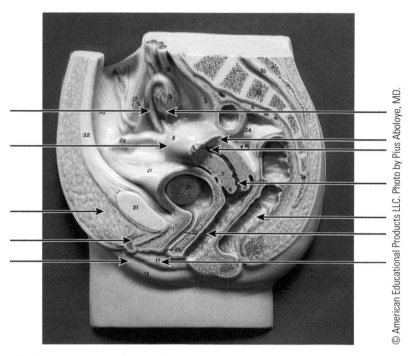

FIGURE 23-10 Female Sagittal View

B.

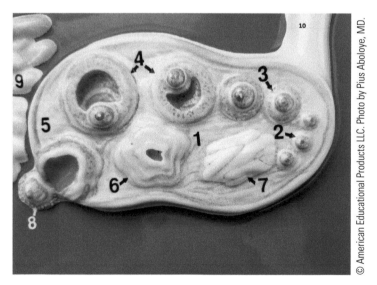

FIGURE 23-11 Female Ovary C/S

See the Photo Atlas

A. Complete the following exercises:

1. Fertilization takes place in the

   A. distal one-third of the fallopian tube

   B. uterus

   C. proximal one-third of the fallopian tube

   D. middle one-third of the fallopian tube

2. During menses in the female

   A. the functional layer of endometrium layer is sloughed off

   B. new secretory glands and blood vessels develop in the endometrium

   C. a new uterine lining is formed

   D. the basal layer of endometrium layer is sloughed off

3. The major hormone produced by the corpus luteum is

   A. estrogen progesterone

   B. FSH

   C. LH

   D. estrogen

4. Define the etiology and signs and symptoms of menopause.

5. List the risk factors for breast cancer.

6. Describe pelvic inflammatory disease (PID) in the female.

7. Distinguish between endometritis and endometriosis.

8. List the three layers of the uterus, from superficial to the deepest layer.

9. List the arterial blood supply to the ovary, uterus, and vagina.

EYE-SAGITTAL VIEW

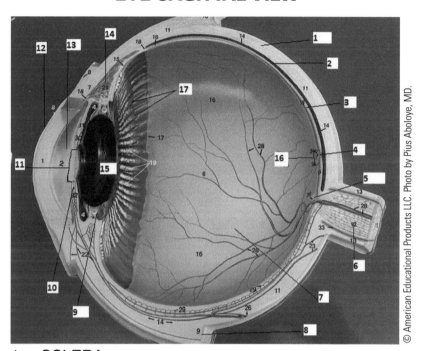

© American Educational Products LLC. Photo by Pius Aboloye, MD.

1. SCLERA
2. CHOROID
3. RETINA
4. MACULA LUTEA
5. OPTIC DISC
6. OPTIC NERVE
7. POSTERIOR CHAMBER (WITH VITREOUS HUMOR)
8. DURA MATER REFLECTION
9. SUSPENSORY LIGAMENT
10. IRIS
11. PUPIL
12. CORNEA
13. ANTERIOR CHAMBER (WITH AQUEOUS HUMOR)
14. CILIARY MUSCLE
15. LENS
16. FOVEA CENTRALIS
17. ORAL SERRATA

EYE MODEL-EXTRINSIC MUSCLES

1. LACRIMAL GLAND
2. LATERAL RECTUS
3. SUPERIOR RECTUS
4. SUPERIOR OBLIQUE
5. INFERIOR OBLIQUE
6. INFERIOR RECTUS

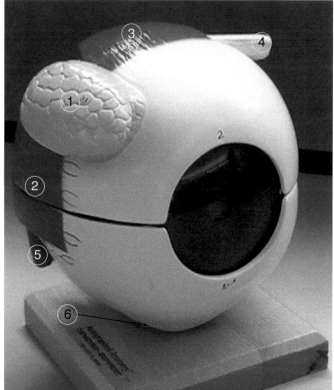

Model manufactured by Denoyer-Geppert. Photo by Pius Aboloye, MD.

EAR MODEL

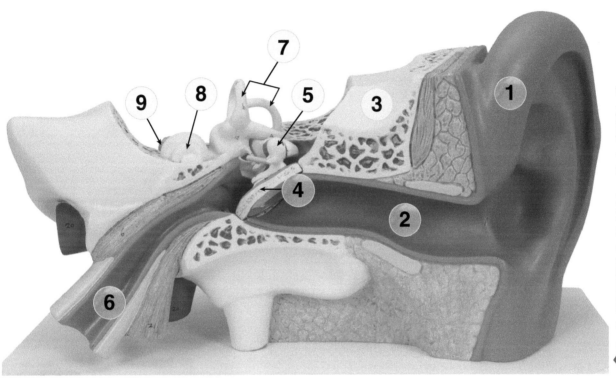

1. PINNAE
2. EXTERNAL AUDITORY MEATUS (CANAL)
3. TEMPORAL BONE
4. TYMPANIC MEMBRANE
5. OSSICLES
6. EUSTACHIAN (PHARYNGOTYMPANIC) TUBE
7. SEMI-CIRCULAR CANALS
8. COCHLEAR
9. VESTIBULOCOCHLEAR N.

EAR OSSICLES

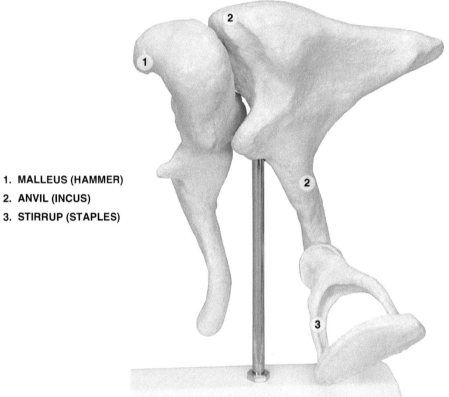

1. MALLEUS (HAMMER)
2. ANVIL (INCUS)
3. STIRRUP (STAPLES)

Item No. 1012786 [A101] - Ossicle Model, 20 times life size, © 3B Scientific GmbH, Germany, 2018, www.3bscientific.com.

BONY LABRYNTH

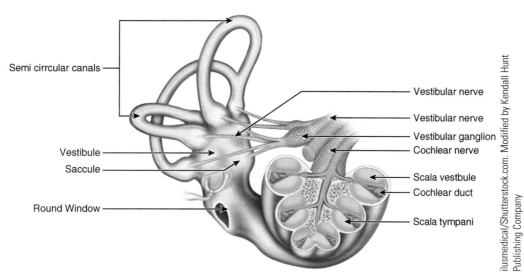

Semi cirrcular canals

Vestibular nerve

Vestibular nerve

Vestibular ganglion

Vestibule

Cochlear nerve

Saccule

Scala vestbule

Cochlear duct

Round Window

Scala tympani

ilusmedical/Shutterstock.com. Modified by Kendall Hunt Publishing Company

COCHLEAR

Scale Vestibule

Cochlear duct

Scale tympani

Cochlear nerve

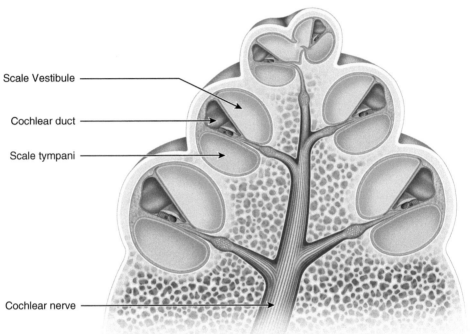

ilusmedical/Shutterstock.com. Modified by Kendall Hunt Publishing Company.

COCHLEAR-MEMBRANOUS LABRYNTH

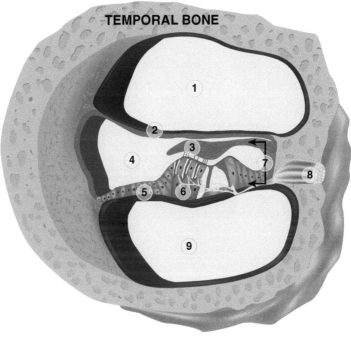

TEMPORAL BONE

1. SCALA VESTIBULE
2. VESTIBULAR MEMBRANE
3. TECTORIAL MEMBRANE
4. COCHLEAR DUCT
5. BASILAR MEMBRANE
6. HAIRY CELLS
7. ORGAN OF CORTI
8. COCHLEAR NERVE
9. SCALA TYMPANI

Sakura/Hunt Publishing Company.

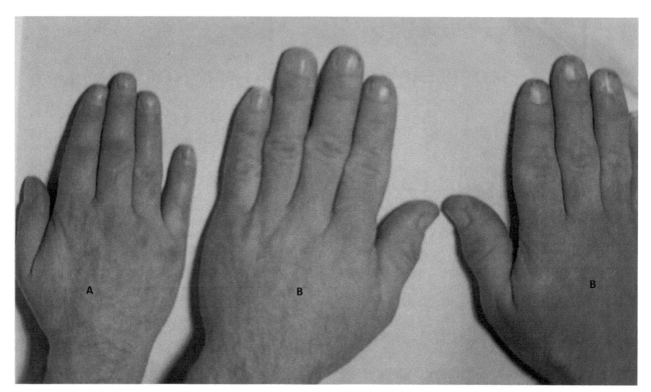

A: NORMAL HAND   VS   B: ACROMEGALY (EXCESS GROWTH HORMONE (ADULT)

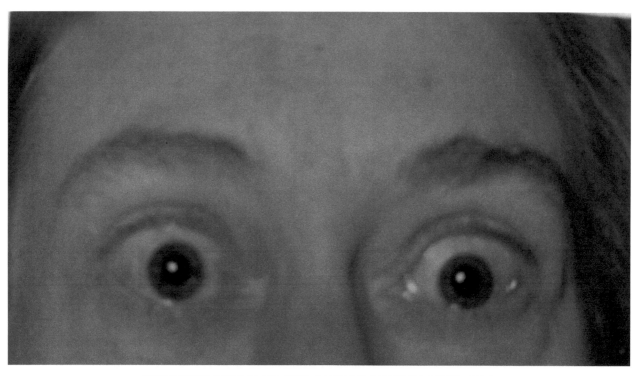

EXOPHTHALMOS IN GRAVES DISEASE (HYPERTHYROIDISM)

HEART BLOOD VESSELS

1. ASCENDING AORTA
2. AORTIC ARCH
3. BRACHIOCEPHALIC TRUNK (ARTERY)
4. L. COMMON CAROTID ARTERY
5. L. SUBCLAVIAN ARTERY
6. PULMONARY TRUNK (ARTERY)
7. SUPERIOR VENA CAVAE (SVC)
8. R. & L. AURICLES
9. R. & L. VENTRICLES
10. LEFT ANTERIOR DESCENDING ARTERY
    (LAD)/ANTERIOR INTERVENTRICULAR
    ARTERY
11. GREAT CARDIAC VEIN

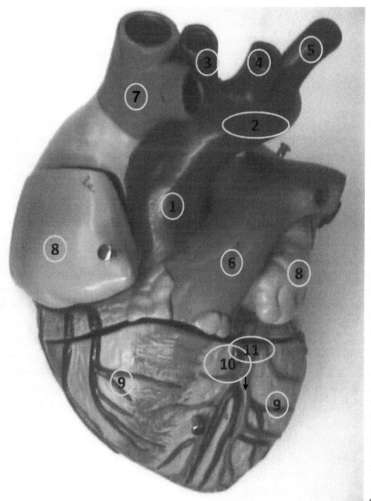

Item No. 1000268 [G12] - Leart, 2-times life size, © 3B Scientific GmbH, Germany, 2018, www.3bscientific.com.
Photo by Pius Aboloye, MD.

HEART: POSTERIOR VIEW

1. **DESCENDING AORTA**
2. **SUPERIOR VENA CAVAE (SVC)**
3. **INFERIOR VENA CAVAE (IVC)**
4. **R. & L. PULMONARY ARTERY**
5. **R. & L. PULMONARY VEINS**
6. **R. &. L. ATRIUM**
7. **R. & L. VENTRICLES**
8. **R. CORONARY ARTERY**
9. **POSTERIOR INTERVENTRICULAR ARTERY**
10. **CORONARY SINUS**

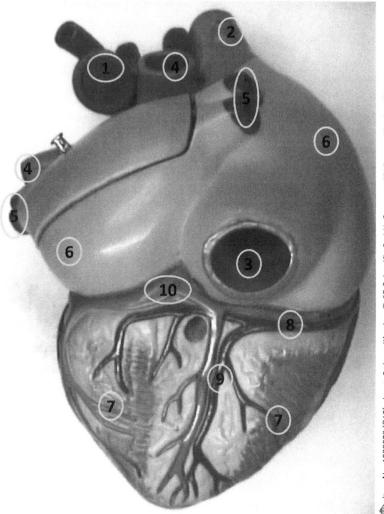

Item No. 1000268 [G12] - Leart, 2-times life size, © 3B Scientific GmbH, Germany, 2018, www.3bscientific.com.

Photo by Pius Aboloye, MD.

HEART INTERNAL STRUCTURES

1. R. ATRIUM
2. PULMONARY VALVES
3. ASCENDING AORTA
4. PULMONARY TRUNK
5. L. ATRIUM
6. BICUSPID (MITRAL) VALVES
7. CHORDAE TENDINEAE
8. TRICUSPID VALVE
9. PAPILLARY MUSCLES
10. R. VENTRICLE
11. L. VENTRICLE
12. INTERVENTRICULAR SEPTUM
13. APEX
14. L. PULMONARY VEINS
15. LIGAMENTUM ARTERIOSUM
16. ARCH OF AORTA
17. SUPERIOR VENA CAVA (SVC)
18. BRACHIOCEPHALIC TRUNK (ARTERY)
19. L. COMMON CAROTID A.
20. L. SUBCLAVIAN A.
21. DESCENDING AORTA
22. R. CORONARY ARTERY
23. L. CORONARY ARTERY

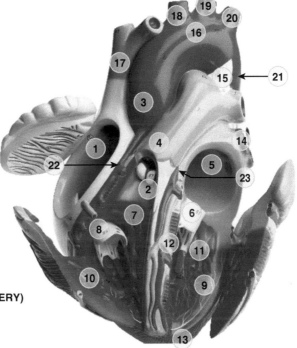

Model manufactured by Denoyer-Geppert. Photo by Pius Aboloye, MD.

BRAIN ARTERIAL SUPPLY VENTRAL VIEW

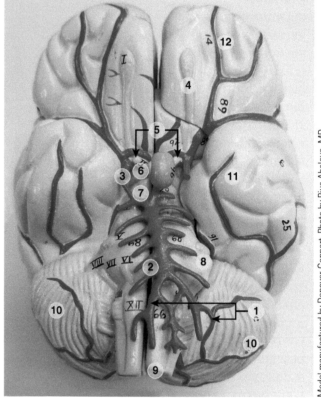

1. R. & L. VERTEBRA ARTERIES
2. BASILAR ARTERY
3. R. INTERNAL CAROTID ARTERIES
4. OLFACTORY NERVE (CN I)
5. OPTIC NERVE (CN II)
6. OPTIC CHIASMA
7. MIDBRAIN
8. PONS
9. MEDULLA OBLONGATA
10. CEREBELLUM
11. TEMPORAL LOBE
12. FRONTAL LOBE

Model manufactured by Denoyer-Geppert. Photo by Pius Aboloye, MD.

HEART WITH MAJOR ARTERIES

1. PULMONARY TRUNK
2. ASCENDING AORTA
3. ARCH OF AORTA
4. LEFT ANTERIOR DESCENDING (LAD)
5. BRACHIOCEPHALIC TRUNK
6. R. & L. COMMON CAROTID ARTERY
7. L. SUBCLAVIAN ARTERY
8. R. SUBCLAVIAN ARTERY
9. SUPERIOR VENA CAVA
10. PULMONARY VESSELS BRANCHES
11. R. & L. ATRIA
12. R. & L. VENTRICLES

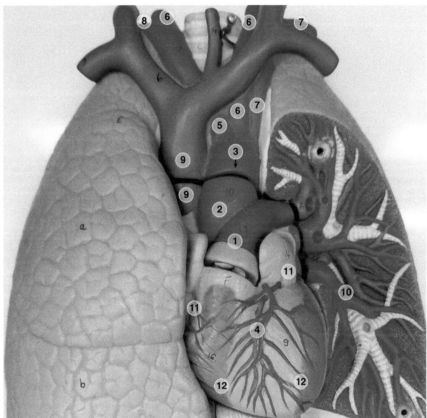

Item No. 1000270 [G15] - Lung model with larynx, © 3B Scientific GmbH, Germany, 2018, www.3bscientific.com. Photo by Pius Aboloye, MD.

HEART WITH MAJOR VEINS

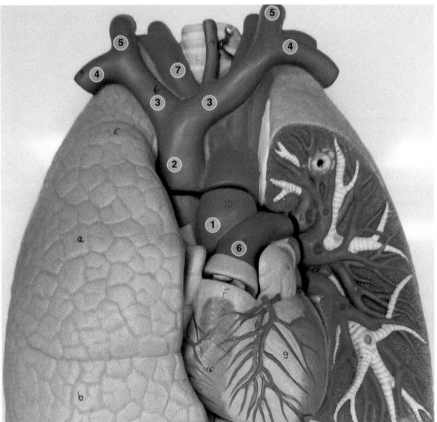

1. AORTA
2. SUPERIOR VENA CAVA
3. R. & L. BRACHIOCEPHALIC VEINS
4. R. & L. SUBCLAVIAN VEINS
5. R. & L. INTERNAL JUGULAR VEINS
6. L. COMMON CAROTID ARTERY
7. BRACHIOCEPHALIC TRUNK (ARTERY)

BLOOD VESSELS-UPPER EXTREMITY-1

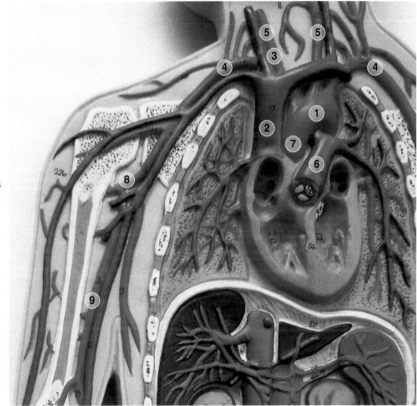

1. AORTIC ARCH
2. SUPERIOR VENA CAVA (SVC)
3. BRACHIOCEPHALIC TRUNK
4. R. & L. SUBCLAVIAN ARTERIES
5. R. & L. COMMON CAROTID A.
6. PULMONARY TRUNK
7. ASCENDING AORTA
8. R. AXILLARY ARTERY
9. R. BRACHIAL ARTERY

BLOOD VESSELS-UPPER EXTREMITY-2
(AND UPPER TRUNK)

1. AORTICARCH
2. SUPERIOR VENA CAVA (SVC)
3. R. & I. BRACHIOCEPHALIC VEINS
4. R. & L. INTERNAL JUGULAR VEINS
5. L. COMMON CAROTID ARTERY
6. L. SUBCLAVIAN ARTERY
7. PULMONARY TRUNK
8. R. BRACHIAL ARTERY
9. R. RADIAL ARTERY
10. R. ULNA ARTERY
11. R. CEPHALIC VEIN
12. R. BASILIC VEIN
13. ABDOMINAL AORTA
14. IINFERIOR VENA CAVA (IVC)
15. R. & L. COMMONILIAC ARTERIES
16. R. & L. EXTERNAL ILIAC ARTERIES

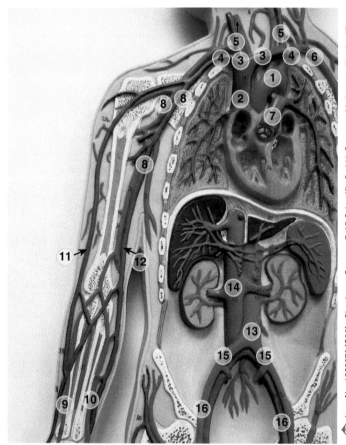

Item No. 1000276 [G30] - Circulatory System, © 3B Scientific GmbH, Germany, 2018, www.3bscientific.com.
Photo by Pius Aboloye, MD.

MAJOR BLOOD VESSELS-RIGHT ARM AND LOWER TRUNK

1. R. BRACHIAL ARTERY
2. R. RADIAL ARTERY & VEIN
3. R. ULNA ARTERY
4. R. BASILIC VEIN
5. R. CEPHALIC VEIN
6. R. RENAL ARTERY & VEIN
7. ABDOMINAL AORTA
8. INFERIOR VENA CAVA (IVC)
9. L. GONADAL ARTERY
10. R. COMMON ILIAC ARTERY & VEIN
11. R. INTERNAL ILIAC ARTERY & VEIN
12. R. EXTERNAL ILIAC ARTERY & VEIN
13. R. FEMORAL ARTERY & VEIN
14. R. GREAT SAPHENOUS VEIN
15. R. PALMAR ARCH ARTERY & VEIN

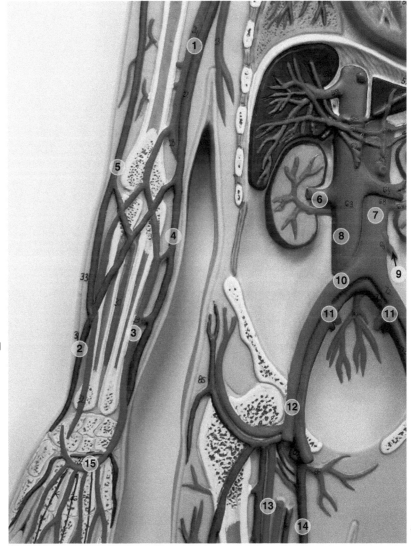

Item No. 1000276 [G30] - Circulatory System, © 3B Scientific GmbH, Germany, 2018, www.3bscientific.com.
Photo by Pius Aboloye, MD.

MAJOR BLOOD VESSELS-LOWER EXTREMITIES

1. L. FEMORAL ARTERY

2. L. POPLITEAL ARTERY

3. L. POSTERIOR TIBIAL ARTERY

4. R. & L. ANTERIOR TIBIAL ARTERY

5. R. & L. DORSAL PEDIS ARTERIES

6. R. GREAT SAPHENOUS VEIN

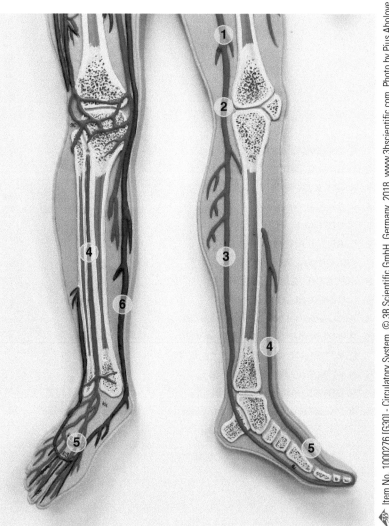

Item No. 1000276 [G30] - Circulatory System, © 3B Scientific GmbH, Germany, 2018, www.3bscientific.com. Photo by Pius Aboloye, MD.

ABDOMINAL PELVIS

1. ILIAC CREST RIGHT
2. ILIACUS
3. PSOAS MAJOR R & L
4. LEFT ILIOPSOAS
5. INGUINAL LIGAMENT LEFT
6. SIGMOID COLON
7. RECTUM
8. BLADDER
9. L. FEMORAL NERVE
10. RIGHT SARTORUS
11. PENIS

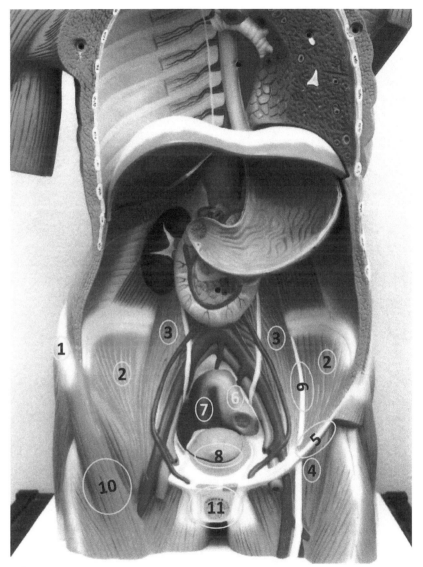

Item No. 1001236 [VA16] - Life size Muscle Torso Model, © 3B Scientific GmbH, Germany, 2018, www.3bscientific.com. Photo by Pius Aboloye, MD.

LYMPHATIC SYSTEM

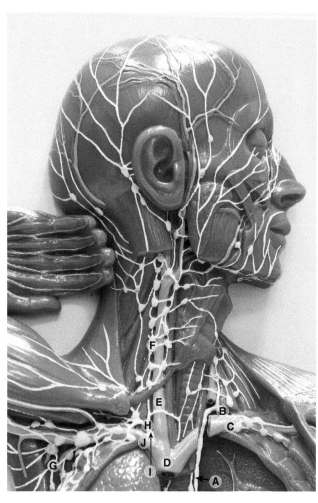

A. THORACIC DUCT

B. THORACIC DUCT OPENING

C. SUBCLAVIAN VEIN LEFT

D. SUPERIOR VENA CAVA

E. INTERNAL JUGULAR VEIN

F. CERVICAL NODES

G. AXILLARY NODES

H. RIGHT LYMPHATIC DUCT

I. RIGHT LYMPHATIC DUCT OPENING

LYMPHATIC SYSTEM

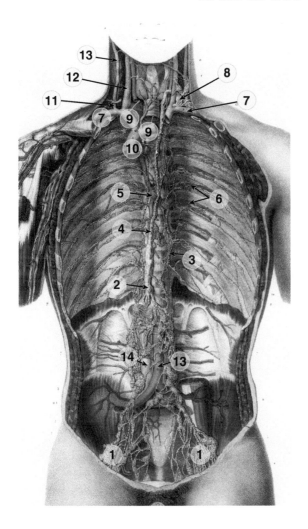

1. PELVIC/INGUINAL LYMPH NODES

2. CYSTERNA CHYLI

3. HEMIAZYGOS VEIN

4. THORACIC DUCT

5. AZYGOS VEIN

6. POSTERIOR INTERCOSTAL VESSELS

7. SUBCLAVIAN VEINS (R/L)

8. THORACIC DUCT OPENING
   (INTO L. SUBCLAVIAN VEIN)

9. BRACHIOCEPHALIC VEINS R/L

10. SUPERIOR VENA CAVA (SVC)

11. RIGHT LYMPHATIC DUCT
    (OPENING INTO R. SUBCLAVIAN VEIN)

12. INTERNAL JUGULAR VEIN R.

13. AORTA (ABDOMINAL)

14. INFERIOR VENA CAVA (IVC)

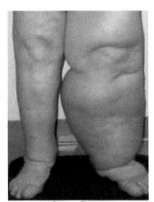

Lymphedema

VENTRAL CAVITY WITH THORACIC DIGESTIVE STRUCTURES

1. R. & L. SUPERIOR LOBES
2. R. & L. OBLIQUE FISSURES
3. TRANSVERSE FISSURE
4. R. MIDDLE LOBE
5. R. & L. LOWER LOBES
6. PERICARDIAC CAVITY
7. DIAPHRAGM
8. LIVER
9. STOMACH
10. TRANSVERSE COLON
11. GREATER OMENTUM
12. SMALL INTESTINE

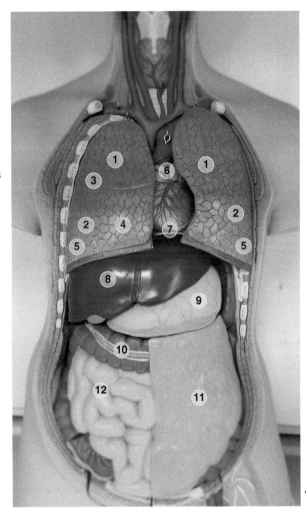

Item No. 1000190 [B13] - Classic Unisex Torso, © 3B Scientific GmbH, Germany, 2018, www.3bscientific.com. Photo by Pius Aboloye, MD.

LUNG ANTERIOR

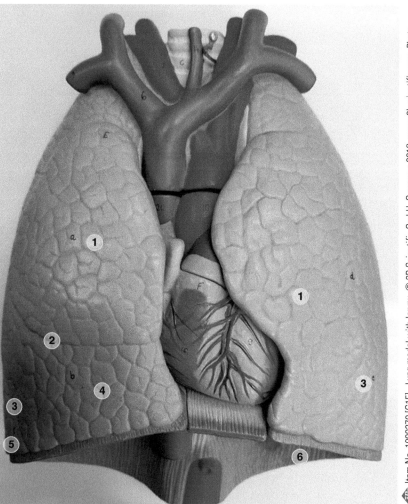

1. R. & L. UPPER LOBES
2. TRANSVERSE/HORIZONTAL FISSURE
3. R. & L. OBLIQUE FISSURES
4. R. MIDDLE LOBE
5. R. INFERIOR LOBE
6. DIAPHRAGRM

Item No. 1000270 [G15] - Lung model with larynx, © 3B Scientific GmbH, Germany, 2018, www.3bscientific.com. Photo by Pius Aboloye, MD.

LUNG FRONTAL VIEW

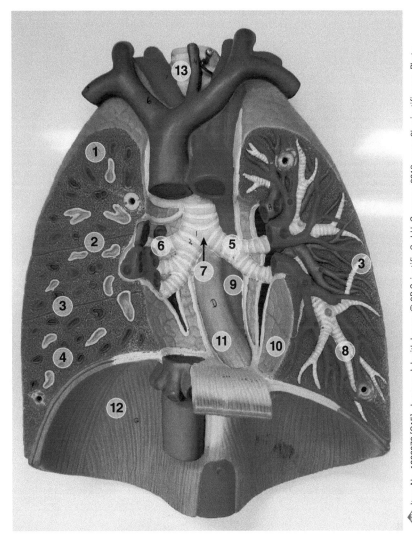

1. UPPER LOBE

2. HORIZONTAL FISSURE

3. R. & L. OBLIQUE FISSURES

4. R. LOWER LOBE

5. L. PRIMARY BRONCHUS

6. R. SECONDARY (LOBAR) BRONCHUS

7. CARINA

8. L. TERTIARY BRONCHII

9. THORACIC AORTA

10. CARDIAC NOTCH

11. ESOPHAGUS

12. DIAPHRAGM

13. TRACHAE

Item No. 1000270 [G15] - Lung model with larynx, © 3B Scientific GmbH, Germany, 2018, www.3bscientific.com. Photo by Pius Aboloye, MD.

LARYNX ANTERIOR VIEW

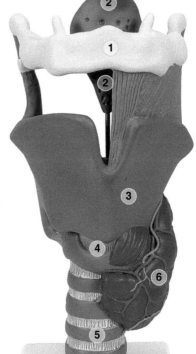

1. HYOID
2. EPIGLOTTIS
3. THROID CARTILAGE
4. CRICO-THYROID MEMBRANE
5. TRACHAE
6. THROID GLAND

Item No. 1013870 [G20] - Functional Larynx Model, © 3B Scientific GmbH, Germany, 2018, www.3bscientific.com.

LARYNX POSTERIOR VIEW

1. EPIGLOTTIS
2. GLOTTIS
3. ARYTENOID CARTILAGE
4. THYROID CARTILAGE
5. THYROID GLAND

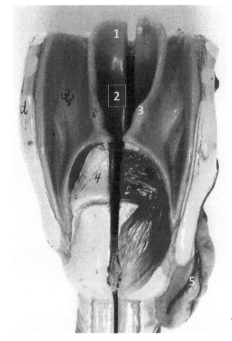

Item No. 1000272 [G21] - Larynx Model, 2 times full-size, © 3B Scientific GmbH, Germany, 2018, www.3bscientific.com. Photo by Pius Aboloye, MD.

LARYNX SAGITTAL VIEW

1. EPIGLOTTIS
2. VESTIBULAR FOLD/FALSE VOCAL CORD
3. TRUE VOCAL CORD
4. TRACHAE
5. THYROID CARTILAGE
6. CRICOID CARTILAGE
7. CRICOTHYROID MEMBRANE

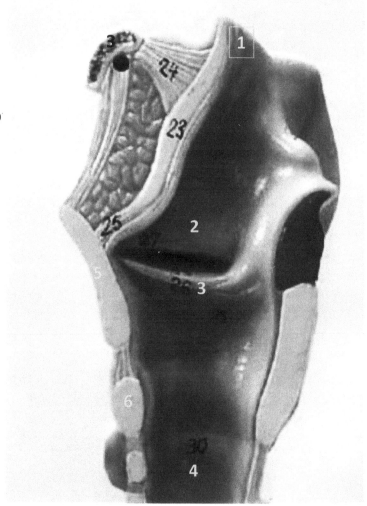

Item No. 1000272 [G21] - Larynx Model, 2 times full-size, © 3B Scientific GmbH, Germany, 2018, www.3bscientific.com. Photo by Pius Aboloye, MD.

THORAX AND UPPER ABDOMIN

1. R. PLEURAL CAVITY
2. L. LUNG
3. L. PRIMARY (MAIN) BRONCHUS
4. L. CARDIAC NOTCH
5. AORTIC ARCH
6. R. PHRENIC NERVE
7. DIAPHRAGM
8. ESOPHAGUS
9. STOMACH
10. GASTROESOPHAGEAL (GE) JUNCTION
11. R. KIDNEY
12. DUODENUM (SMALL INTESTINE)

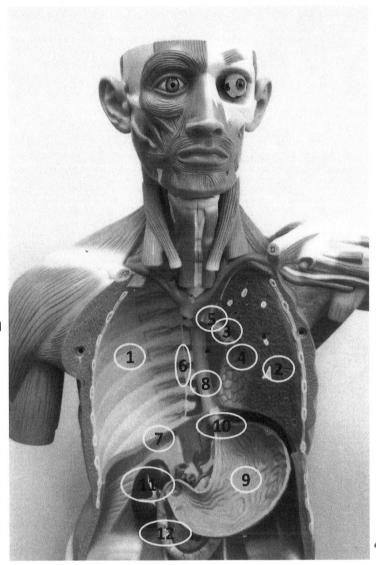

Item No. 1001236 [VA16] - Life size Muscle Torso Model, © 3B Scientific GmbH, Germany, 2018, www.3bscientific.com. Photo by Pius Aboloye, MD.

HEAD-NECK SAGITTAL VIEW

1. SUBLINGUAL GLAND LEFT

2. SUBMANDIBULAR GLAND LEFT

3. LARYNX

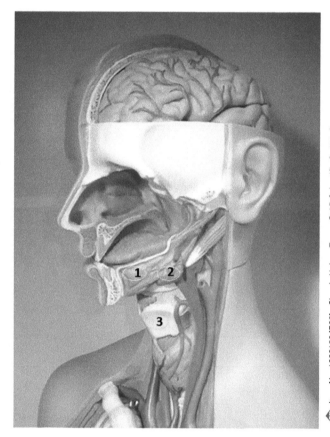

Item No. 1000186 [B09] - Classic Unisex Torso, © 3B Scientific GmbH, Germany, 2018, www.3bscientific.com. Photo by Pius Aboloye, MD.

HEAD-NECK SAGITTAL VIEW

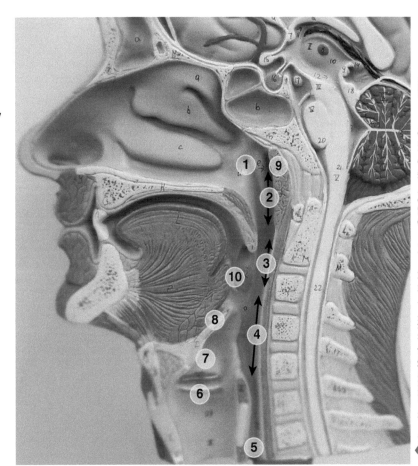

1. OPENINING OF EUSTACHIAN / PHARYNGOTYMPANIC TUBE

2. NASOPHARYNX

3. OROPHARYNX

4. LARYNGOPHARYNX

5. ESOPHAGUS

6. TRUE VOCAL CORD

7. VESTIBULAR FOLD (FALSE VOCAL CORD)

8. EPIGLOTTIS

9. PHARYNGEAL TONSIL

10. PALATINE TONSIL

Item No. 1000221 [C14] - Half Head with Musculature, © 3B Scientific GmbH, Germany, 2018, www.3bscientific.com. Photo by Pius Aboloye, MD.

THORACO-ABDOMINAL STRUCTURES

1. **ESOPHAGUS (WITH VAGUS NERVE PLEXUS)**
2. **DIAPHRAGM**
3. **GASTROESOHAGEAL (GE) JUNCTION**
4. **FUNDUS Of STOMACH**
5. **CIRCULAR MUSCLE (STOMACH)**
6. **BODY OF STOMACH**
7. **DUODENUM**
8. **TRANSVERSE COLON**
9. **R. COLON FLEXURE**

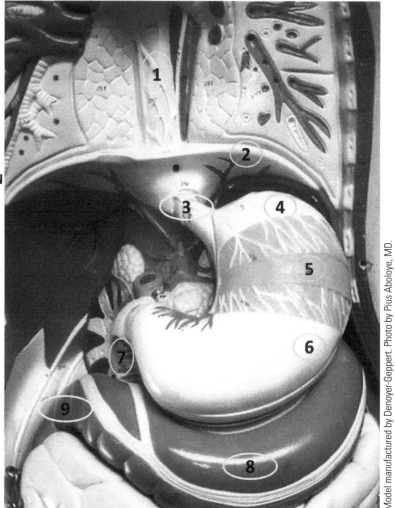

Model manufactured by Denoyer-Geppert. Photo by Pius Aboloye, MD.

GI STRUCTURES
(STOMACH/LIVER/SI REMOVED)

1. DIAPHRAGM
2. CELIAC TRUNK (ARTERY)
3. INFERIOR VENA CAVA
4. R. & L. SUPRARENAL (ADRENAL GLANDS)
5. SPLEEN
6. PANCREAS
7. MAIN PANCREATIC DUCT
8. DUODENUM
9. R. KIDNEY
10. ASCENDING COLON
11. CECUM
12. SIGMOID COLON
13. HAUSTRA
14. DESCENDING COLON
15. JEJUNUM
16. ILEUM TERMINAL
17. MESENTARY /MESOCOLON
18. BLADDER

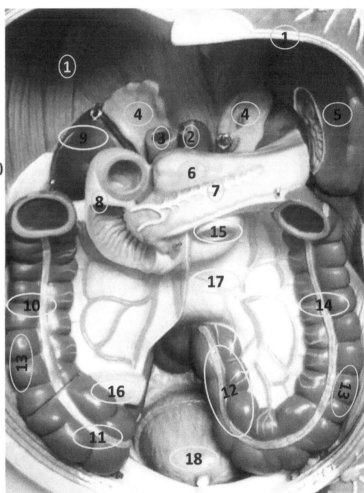

Item No. 1000192 [B17] - Classic Unisex Torso with Open Back, © 3B Scientific GmbH, Germany, 2018, www.3bscientific.com. Photo by Pius Aboloye, MD.

STOMACH

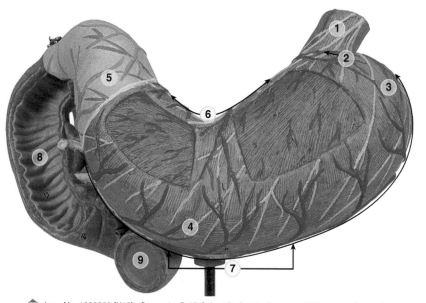

1. ESOPHAGUS
2. GASTROESOHAGEAL (GE) JUNCTION
3. FUNDUS OF STOMACH
4. BODY (STOMACH)
5. PYLORUS REGION OF STOMACH
6. LESSER CURVATURE
7. GREATER CURVATURE
8. DUODENUM
9. JEJUNUM

Item No. 1000303 [K16] - Stomach, © 3B Scientific GmbH, Germany, 2018, www.3bscientific.com.

STOMACH

Posterior Section   ## Frontal Section

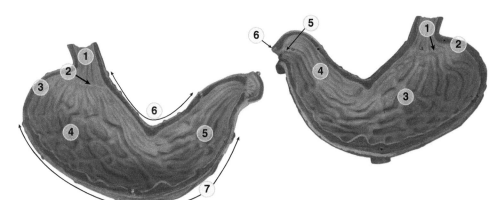

Item No. 1000303 [K16] - Stomach, © 3B Scientific GmbH, Germany, 2018, www.3bscientific.com.

1. ESOPHAGUS
2. GASTROESOPHAGEAL (GE) JUNCTION
3. FUNDUS OF STOMACH
4. BODY (STOMACH)
5. PYLORUS REGION OF STOMACH
6. LESSER CURVATURE
7. GREATER CURVATURE

1. GASTROESOPHAGEAL (GE) SPHINCTER
2. FUNDUS OF STOMACH
3. RUGAE (STOMACH) MUCOSA FOLDS
4. PYLORUS REGION OF STOMACH
5. PYLORUS SPHINCTER
6. DUODENUM

LIVER ANTERIOR

CORONARY
LIGAMENT

RIGHT LOBE

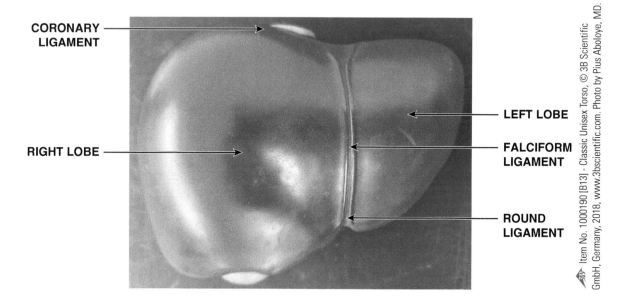

LEFT LOBE

FALCIFORM
LIGAMENT

ROUND
LIGAMENT

Item No. 1000190 [B13] - Classic Unisex Torso, © 3B Scientific GmbH, Germany, 2018, www.3bscientific.com. Photo by Pius Aboloye, MD.

LIVER POSTERIOR

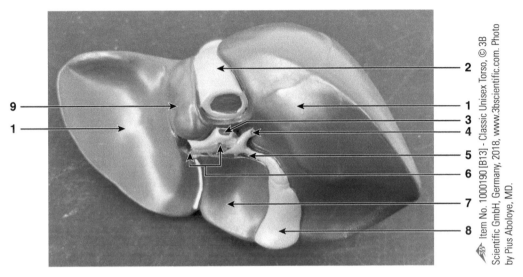

1. LEFT LOBE
2. INFERIOR VENA CAVA
3. HEPATIC PORTAL VEIN
4. COMMON BILE DUCT
5. CYSTIC DUCT
6. HEPATIC ARTERIES
7. CAUDATE LOBE
8. GALLBLADDER
9. QUADRATE LOBE

HEPATO-BILIARY TRACK

1. SPLEEN
2. PANCREAS TAIL
3. MAIN PANCREATIC DUCT
4. DUODENUM
5. HEPATOPANCREATIC AMPULLA
6. SUPERIOR MESENTERIC ARTERY & VEIN
7. JEJUNUM
8. CYST DUCT
9. COMMON BILE DUCT
10. HEPATIC DUCT
11. HEPATIC ARTERY AND VEIN
12. STOMACH (CUT)

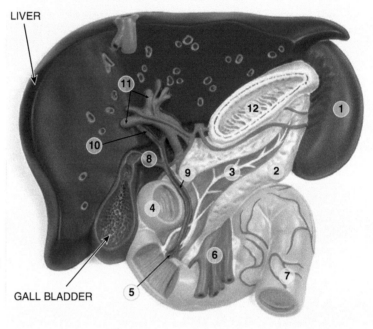

LIVER

GALL BLADDER

Item No. 1008550 [VE315] - Liver with Gall Bladder, Pancreas and Duodenum, © 3B Scientific GmbH, Germany, 2018, www.3bscientific.com.

PANCREAS ANTERIOR

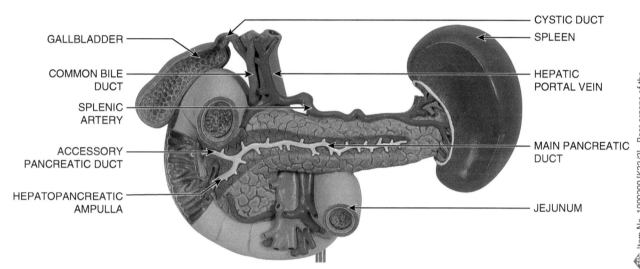

GALLBLADDER

COMMON BILE
DUCT

SPLENIC
ARTERY

ACCESSORY
PANCREATIC DUCT

HEPATOPANCREATIC
AMPULLA

CYSTIC DUCT

SPLEEN

HEPATIC
PORTAL VEIN

MAIN PANCREATIC
DUCT

JEJUNUM

Item No. 1000309 [K22/2] - Rear organs of the upper abdomen, © 3B Scientific GmbH, Germany, 2018, www.3bscientific.com.

PANCREAS POSTERIOR

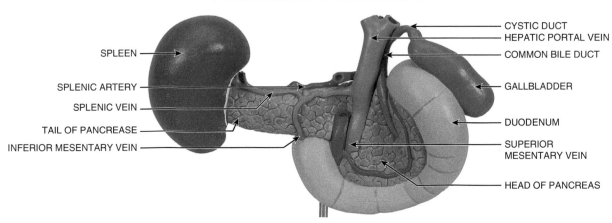

SPLEEN

SPLENIC ARTERY

SPLENIC VEIN

TAIL OF PANCREASE

INFERIOR MESENTARY VEIN

CYSTIC DUCT
HEPATIC PORTAL VEIN
COMMON BILE DUCT

GALLBLADDER

DUODENUM

SUPERIOR
MESENTARY VEIN

HEAD OF PANCREAS

Item No. 1000309 [K22/2] - Rear organs of the upper abdomen, © 3B Scientific GmbH, Germany, 2018, www.3bscientific.com.

PANCREAS-DUODENUM-SPLEEN

1. DUODENUM
2. MINOR PANCREATIC DUCT
3. MAIN PANCREATIC DUCT
4. SPLENIC ARTERY
5. SPLEEN
6. PANCREAS
7. JEJUNUM
8. SUPERIOR MESENTERIC ARTERY & VEIN
9. PLICAE CIRCULARIS (CIRCULAR FOLDS)
10. DUODENAL PAPILLA
11. COMMON BILE DUCT

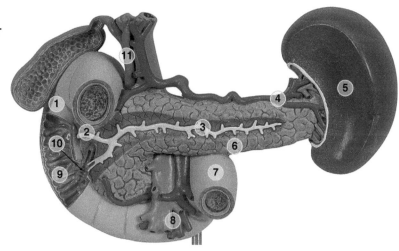

Item No. 1000309 [K22/2] - Rear organs of the upper abdomen, © 3B Scientific GmbH, Germany, 2018, www.3bscientific.com.

COLON-1

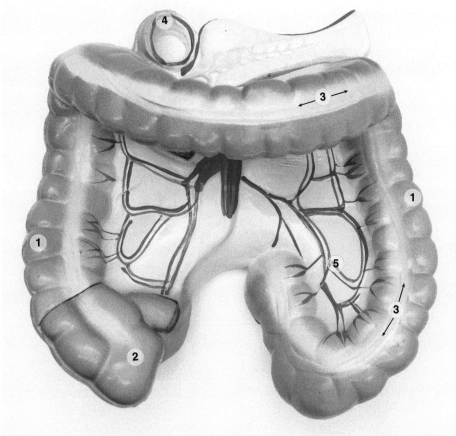

1. **HAUSTRA**
2. **CECUM**
3. **TEANIA COLI (MUSCLE)**
4. **DUODENUM**
5. **MESENTERY WITH BLOOD VESSELS**

Bangkoker/Shutterstock.com. Modified by Kendall Hunt Publishing Company

SMALL INTESTIONAL WALL

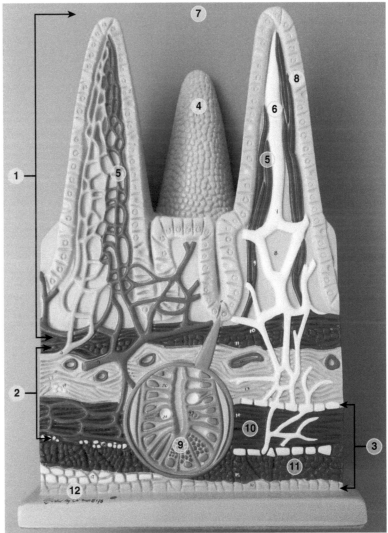

1. MUCOSA
2. SUBMUCOSA
3. MUSCULARIS EXTERNAL
4. VILLI
5. CAPILLARY & VENULES
6. LACTEAL
7. GI LUMEN
8. VILLI EPITHELIUM (COLUMNAR)
9. PEYERS PATCHES (LYMPH NODULE)
10. CIRCULAR MUSCLE
11. LONGITUDINAL MUSCLE
12. SEROSA

Model manufactured by Denoyer-Geppert. Photo by Pius Aboloye, MD.

COLON-2

COLON-2

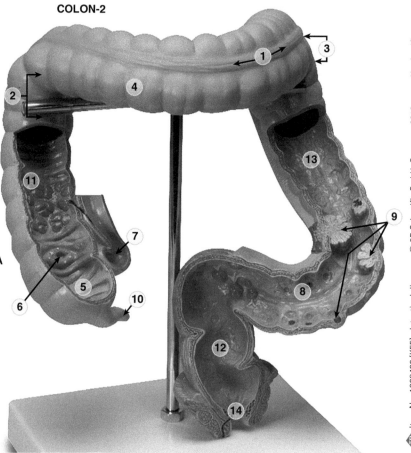

1. TENIA COLI
2. R. COLON (HEPATIC) FLEXURE
3. L. COLON (SPLENIC) FLEXURE
4. TRANSVERSE COLON
5. CECUM
6. ILEOCECAL VALVE/JUNCTION
7. ILEUM TERMINAL
8. SIGMOID COLON
9. DISEASED COLON WITH DIVERTICULA
10. APPENDIX
11. ASCENDING COLON
12. RECTUM
13. DESCENDING COLON
14. ANUS

KUB STAND-FRONTAL VIEW

1. R. & L. KIDNEYS

2. R. & L. ADRENAL GLANDS

3. R. & L. RENAL ARTERIES & VEINS

4. URETERS

5. R. & L. COMMON ILIAC ARTERIES & VEINS

6. INFERIOR VENA CAVA

7. AORTA (ABDOMINAL)

8. CELIAC TRUNK

9. SUPERIOR MESSENTARY ARTERY (SMA)

10. R. GONADAL ARTERY

11. INFERIOR MESSENTARY ARTERY (IMA)

12. BLADDER

13. PUBIC SYMPHYSIS

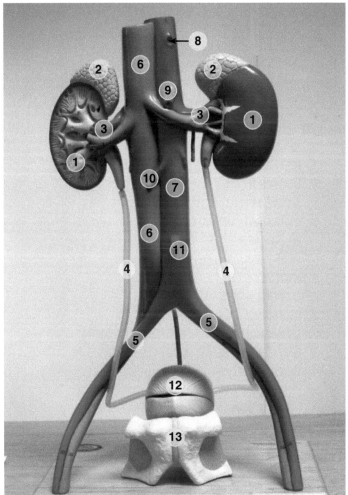

Model manufactured by Denoyer-Geppert. Photo by Pius Aboloye, MD.

URINARY-PELVIS

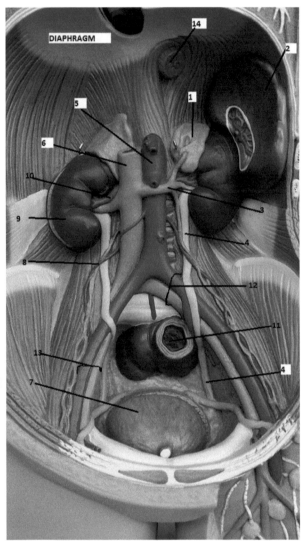

1. ADRENAL GLAND
2. SPLEEN
3. RENAL VEIN
4. URETER
5. ABDOMINAL AORTA
6. INFERIOR VENA CAVA
7. BLADDER
8. GONADAL ARTERY AND VEIN
9. KIDNEY
10. RENAL ARTERY
11. SIGMOID COLON
12. COMMON ILIAC ARTERY AND VEIN
13. EXTERNAL ILIAC ARTERY AND VEIN
14. ESOPHAGUS

Item No. 1000192 [B17] - Classic Unisex Torso with Open Back, © 3B Scientific GmbH, Germany, 2018, www.3bscientific.com. Photo by Pius Aboloye, MD.

KIDNEY FRONTAL SECTION

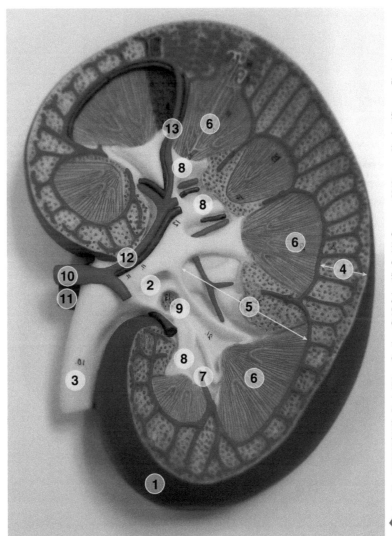

1. RENAL CAPSULE
2. RENAL PELVIS
3. URETER
4. RENAL CORTEX
5. RENAL MEDULLA
6. PYRAMID
7. COLUMN
8. MINOR CALYX
9. MAJOR CALYX
10. RENAL ARTERY
11. RENAL VEIN
12. SEGMENTAL ARTERY
13. INTERLOBAR ARTERY & VEIN

Item No. 1000295 [K09] - Basic Kidney Section, © 3B Scientific GmbH, Germany, 2018, www.3bscientific.com. Photo by Pius Aboloye, MD.

ABDOMINAL PELVIC CAVITY

1. R. KIDNEY
2. PANCREAS (HEAD)
3. DUODENUM
4. R. & L. GONADAL ARTERIES
5. L. URETER
6. R. COMMON ILIAC ARTERY & VEIN
7. L. INTERNAL ILIAC ARTERY & VEIN
8. R. & L. EXTERNAL ILIAC ARTERIES & VEINS
9. R. FEMORAL ARTERY & VEIN
10. L. FEMORAL ARTERY/VEIN & NERVE
11. INGUNAL LIGAMENT
12. DIAPHRAGM
13. STOMACH
14. DUODENUM
15. SIGMOID COLON
16. BLADDER

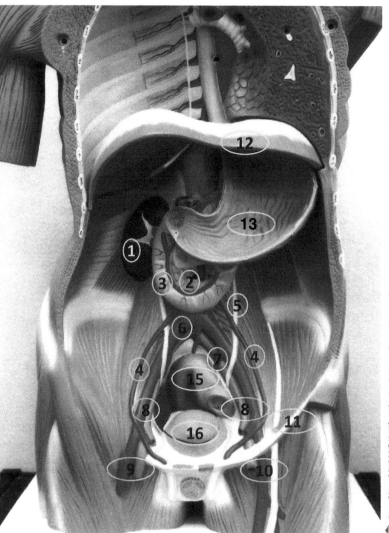

Item No. 1001236 [VA16] - Life size Muscle Torso Model, © 3B Scientific GmbH, Germany, 2018, www.3bscientific.com. Photo by Pius Aboloye, MD.

MAJOR BLOOD VESSELS-ABDOMINAL-PELVIC

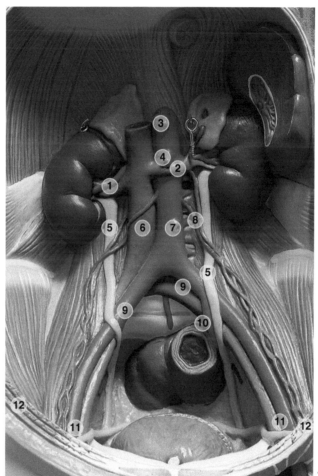

1. R. RENAL ARTERY & VEIN
2. L. RENAL VEIN
3. CELIAC TRUNK (ARTERY)
4. SUPERIOR MESENTERIC ARTERY
5. R. & L. URETERS
6. INFERIOR VENA CAVA (IVC)
7. ABDOMINAL AORTA
8. L. GONADAL ARTERY
9. R. & L. COMMON ILIAC ARTERIES & VEINS
10. R. & L. INTERNAL ILIAC ARTERIES & VEINS
11. R. & L. EXTERNAL ILIAC ARTERIES & VEINS
12. R. & L. INGUINAL LIGAMENT

RENAL LOBULE

1. RENAL CAPSULE
2. RENAL CORTEX
3. RENAL MEDULLA
4. INTERLOBAR ARTERY
5. ARCUATE (CORTICAL RADIATE)
5b. INTERLOBULAR ARTERY
6. GLOMERULUS
7. PROXIMAL CONVOLUTED TUBULE (PCT)
8. DESCENDING LOOP
9. ASCENDING LOOP
10. DISTAL CONVOLUTED TUBULE (DCT)
11. COLLECTING DUCT
12. VASA RECTA (ARTERIES/VEINS)
13. RENAL PAPILLA

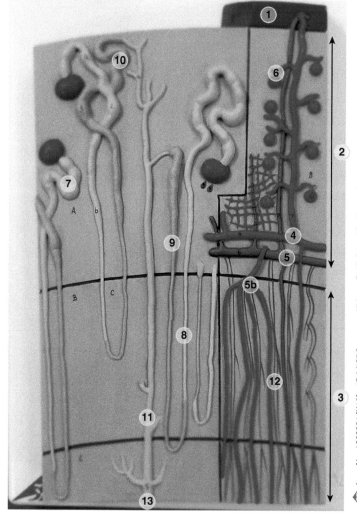

Item No. 1000301 [K13] - #B MICROanatomy Kidney, © 3B Scientific GmbH, Germany, 2018, www.3bscientific.com. Photo by Pius Aboloye, MD.

RENAL CORPUSCLE

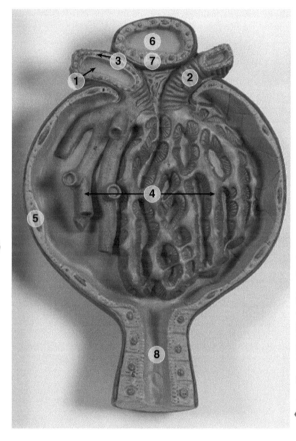

1. AFFERENT ARTERIOLE
2. EFFERENT ARTERIOLE
3. GRANULAR CELLS (AFFERENT)
4. GLOMERULUS CAPILLARY
5. GLOMERULUS CAPSULE
6. DISTAL CONVOLUTED TUBULE (DCT)
7. MACULA DENSA (OF DCT)
8. PROXIMAL CONVOLUTED TUBULE

Item No. 1000299 [K11] - Kidney Section, Nephrons, Blood Vessels and Renal Corpuscle, © 3B Scientific GmbH, Germany, 2018, www.3bscientific.com.

MALE REPRODUCTIVE ANTERIOR VIEW

1. **GLANS PENIS**
2. **TESTIS**
3. **EPIDIDYMUS**
4. **SPERMATIC CORD**
5. **URINARY BLADDER**

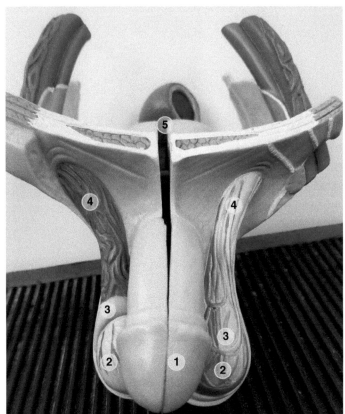

Item No. 1000196 [B30] - Deluxe Dual Sex Torso, © 3B Scientific GmbH, Germany, 2018, www.3bscientific.com. Photo by Pius Aboloye, MD.

MALE REPRODUCTIVE SAGITTAL VIEW

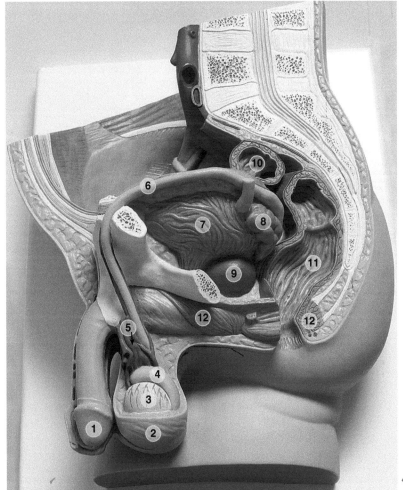

1. GLANS PENIS
2. SCROTAL SAC
3. TESTIS
4. EPIDYDIMUS
5. SPERMATIC CORD
6. VAS DEFERENS
7. URINARY BLADDER
8. SEMINAL VESSICLE GLAND
9. PROSTATE GLAND
10. SIGMOID COLON
11. RECTUM
12. EXTERNAL SPHINCTER
    (PELVIC DIAPHRAGM)

Item No. 1000282 [H11] - Male Pelvis, © 3B Scientific GmbH, Germany, 2018, www.3bscientific.com.

Photo by Pius Aboloye, MD.

MALE REPRODUCTIVE SAGITTAL VIEW

1. CORPUS CARVONOSA (OF PENIS)
2. SPONGY URETHRA (WITHIN CORPUS SPONGIOSUM OF PENIS)
3. EPIDIDYMUS
4. SPERMATIC CORD
5. URINARY BLADDER
6. PROSTATIC URETHRA
7. PROSTATE GLAND
8. EJACULATORY DUCT

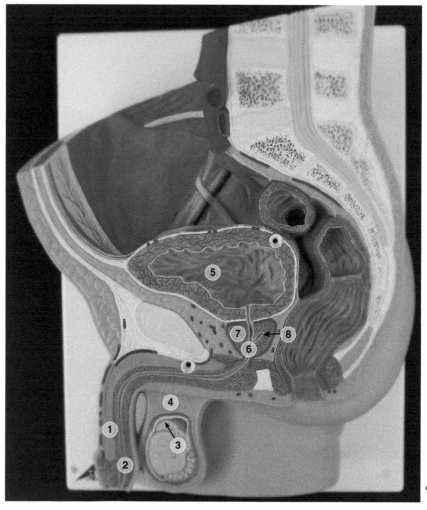

Item No. 1000282 [H11] - Male Pelvis, © 3B Scientific GmbH, Germany, 2018, www.3bscientific.com.
Photo by Pius Aboloye, MD.

FEMALE REPRODUCTIVE SAGITTAL VIEW

1. MONS PUBIS
2. LABIA MAJOR
3. BLADDER
4. URETHRA
5. VAGINA
6. CERVIX
7. RECTUM
8. EXTERNAL SPHINCTER
   (PELVIC DIAPHRAGM)
9. SIGMOID COLON
10. UTERUS
11. FALLOPIAN TUBE

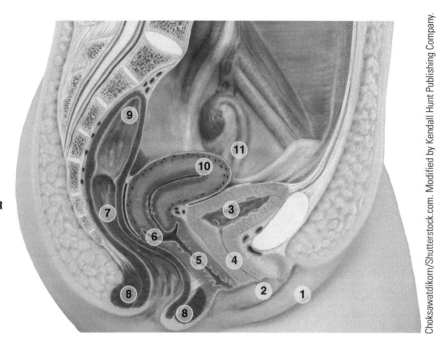

Choksawatdikorn/Shutterstock.com. Modified by Kendall Hunt Publishing Company.

FEMALE REPRODUCTIVE VIEW

1. VAGINA
2. CERVIX
3. CERVICAL CANAL
4. UTERINE CANAL
5. MYOMETRIUM WALL
6. OVARIAN LIGAMENT
7. FALLOPIAN TUBES
8. FIMBRAE
9. OVARY

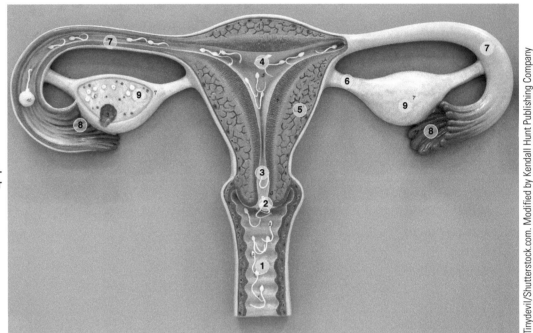

Tinydevil/Shutterstock.com. Modified by Kendall Hunt Publishing Company

FEMALE OVARY CS

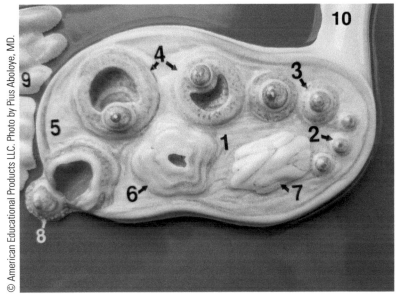

1. MEDULLA/STROMA
2. PRIMARY FOLLICLES
3. SECONDARY FOLLICLES
4. GRAFFIAN FOLLICLES
5. CORTEX
6. CORPUS LUTEUM
7. CORPUS ALBICAN
8. OVULATION (OVUM)
9. PART FIMBRAE
10. OVARIAN LIGAMENT (PART)